Tibetan Medicine
in Contemporary Tibet
Health and Health Care in Tibet II

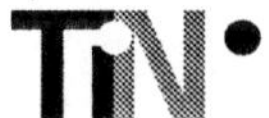

Tibet Information Network

London 2004

Printed in England
Published by Tibet Information Network (TIN), July 2004

Design & Typesetting
Matthew Ward

ISBN: 0-9541961-7-1

Tibetan Medicine in Contemporary Tibet:

Health and Health care in Tibet II

Tibet Information Network (TIN):

UK HEAD OFFICE:

City Cloisters,
188-196 Old Street
London EC1V 9FR UK

tel: +44 (0)20 7814 9011
fax: +44 (0)20 7814 9015

US OFFICE:

TIN USA
PO Box 2270
Jackson WY83001

tel: +1 307 733 4670
fax: +1 307 739 2501

tin@tibetinfo.net — www.tibetinfo.net — tinusa@wyoming.com

TiN •   Tibet Information Network...

culture

economy

education

environment

health

leaders

media

policies

prisoners

propaganda

religion

tourism

women

Tibet Information Network (TIN) is an independent news service and research organisation that gathers and disseminates information about the situation in Tibet. Based in London with field teams in India and Nepal, TIN monitors political, social, economic, environmental, and human rights conditions in Tibet, and then publishes this information in the form of regular news updates (via email and the web), special reports, briefing papers and specialist publications. TIN's information comes from a variety of sources both inside and outside Tibet, official and informal, as well as from its own fieldwork with Tibetan refugees, and from the monitoring of established Chinese, Tibetan and international media.

TIN's primary objective is to provide a systematic, comprehensive and impartial news, research and information service for development agencies, governments, and non-governmental and international organisations, as well as journalists, academics, human rights groups and other interested parties.
Over the last 15 years TIN has gained a worldwide reputation for reliable fact-based reporting and expert analysis of conditions and developments in present-day Tibet.

In 1996 – nine years after it was first established – TIN was registered as a charity in the UK under the title "Tibet Information Network Trust", with the following stated aims:

- *to advance the education of the public about Tibet and its people*
  by undertaking, promoting and commissioning research into
  conditions and developments in and relating to Tibet.

- *to disseminate the results of such research to the general public,*
  non-governmental organisations, inter-governmental organisations,
  governments, parliamentarians, the media and scholars in the UK
  and throughout the world.

Acknowledgements

TIN would not have been able to compile this report without the assistance of many people and institutions.

Our particular gratitude goes to **Lawrie Plantation Services** and the **Camellia Foundation** who generously financed this book project.

We would also like to thank all donors who supported TIN's operations during the time this publication was prepared, in particular, the Barrow Cadbury Trust; Heinrich Böll Stiftung; the Isdell 86 Foundation; David Lacey; the National Endowment for Democracy; the Ruben & Elisabeth Rausing Trust; the Sigrid Rausing Trust; the Stahl Family Foundation; the Staples Trust; the Swedish International Development Cooperation Agency (SIDA); and Swedish Amnesty Fund; as well as many other donors all over the world, some of whom have preferred to remain anonymous.

Though all of them cannot be listed here, TIN is also thankful to many persons who in one way or the other contributed to make this publication possible, in particular Amber Cripps, Jean-Marc Dodin, Dickyi Lhamo, Stuart Wright, and a great number other contributors, advisors, supporters, interns and volunteers.

Last but not least, we would like to thank those Tibetans who had the patience to answer our questions and share their experiences and insights with us. Without their contribution writing this book would have been obviously impossible.

Contents

A Note on the Use of Tibetan Terms and Concepts

Throughout the text, we have chosen to represent Tibetan spellings phonetically, as opposed to transliterating them using the established Wylie system. We have done this to ease the reader's comprehension and ability to pronounce non-English terms. However, we have provided a glossary that details the phonetic spellings, the Wylie transliterations, and an English translation for these terms and concepts. In addition, and in order to facilitate the reader's understanding, we have provided several charts, graphs, and illustrations when describing some of the more intricate Tibetan medical concepts.

A Note on Bibliographic Sources and Citations

We have tried to make this text both reflective of and informed by the scholarship on Tibetan medicine and at the same time accessible to the lay reader. As a result, instead of including many footnotes and references within the text itself, we have provided a bibliography as well as a suggested reading list at the end of the book. The bibliography includes both references for direct citations that do appear in footnotes, as well as other scholarly articles and books that have informed the writing of this text. The list of suggested reading on Tibetan medicine is geared primarily toward the non-specialist, and is intended to provide an approachable overview of the subject. In addition, where we have compiled and condensed a number of scholarly works on a given topic, such as the history of Tibetan medicine given in Chapter One, we have listed several of the key authors in such areas in a footnote at the beginning of the section or chapter.

O Transcendent Conqueror, Healer King of Physicians, O Medicine Guru Buddha, who dispels afflictions of the three poisons, whose indigo form emits aquamarine light, and whose emanated body is endowed with the major and minor marks; in your right hand you hold a chebulic myrobalan, the antidote to the afflictions of those who are tormented by disorders of wind, bile, and phlegm. I prostrate to the one who emits aquamarine light and who holds in his left hand a begging bowl filled with nectar. He has realised the eighteen supreme sciences and has attained the powerful attainment of essence-extraction, which brings mastery over life itself. I prostrate to the Rishi Vidhyadhara, the Supreme Being who balanced collective imbalances of the bodily humours, and who is endowed with clairvoyance and compassion. To the gods this medicine is like nectar, to the serpent spirits like a crowning jewel and to the sages like the essence-extraction pills. May it subdue the four hundred and four diseases of wind, bile, and phlegm, which threaten life, also subdue the one thousand and eighty types of harmful interferences, the three hundred and sixty intrinsic spirits, and mental obstacles.

    – From 'The Healer Physician,' Chapter 31 of the Explanatory Tantra (*Chima Gyu*) of the Four Medical Tantras (*Gyushi*)

After Tibet's peaceful liberation, especially since reforming and widening the support of and paying serious attention to the Communist Party and the Government, traditional Tibetan medicine has been developed as a centre of Tibetan medical treatment, teaching, and scientific research…Famous ancient Tibetan medicine and remarkably talented persons are gathered here [at the Lhasa Mentsikhang]. Thus, it is the highest institution of Tibetan medicine, as they say, a "cloud of talented scholars"…For the treatment of common diseases, uncommon diseases, and diversified diseases, the special treatment methods of Tibetan medicine and natural medicine materials of Tibet's plateau are used…In the light of the great efforts of staff members of [the Mentsikhang]…Tibetan medicine has been developed. It is not only trusted by Tibetans, but each nationality of the State as well. Moreover, it will be receiving honours from all corners of the world.

    – From the Tibetan Pharmaceutical Factory of the Tibet Medical Hospital of the TAR [Mentsikhang] brochure

"It is not a problem to make money. The problem is how we make the medicines now, what the ingredients are like, how they are collected. Before, we prepared medicines by first harvesting the ingredients well – taking care with the time we collect, the tastes of the medicines, how much we take when, the nature of our minds when we collected. Then we mixed the ingredients together and ground them by hand. If you read the texts, there are even different descriptions of how your body should feel – where you should be in pain – after making medicines. But now, from Beijing and other parts in China and the world that buy our medicine, they tell us that each ingredient has to be clean, and that you should mix the medicines in these big machines. But what do they mean by 'clean'? It is different than how we have been taught to make medicines. Now they even make new kind of rilbu, *that aren't really* rilbu. *They call them 'capsule.' They are strange, but they say they're cleaner. They look like western medicine. We make a lot of them."*

    – A Tibetan doctor in contemporary Lhasa

Summary Points

This TIN book examines the relationship between Tibetan medicine and contemporary Tibetan society. We are concerned with the perpetuation of Tibetan medicine in today's Tibet, as well as its future prospects as a science, healing art, an affordable and available component of the health care systems at work in Tibet, and an indicator of cultural, linguistic, and religious survival. Below are several key points that summarise issues covered in this book.

- Tibetan medicine has been practiced throughout the Tibetan Plateau, Himalayas, and Central Asia since at least the seventh century. In addition to its historical legacy and current importance among Tibetan communities within the PRC, Tibetan medicine is practiced in other parts of South, East, and Central Asia, from Ladakh, Spiti, and Sikkim in India, to northern Nepal, Bhutan, Mongolia, and Buryatia.

- Tibetan medicine is fundamentally connected with Tibetan Buddhism: Sangye Menla, the 'Medicine Buddha', is viewed as the source of medical teachings and the inspiration for correct practice as a physician.

- The annexation of Tibet by the People's Republic of China (PRC) in the 1950s and the subsequent Tibetan diaspora have greatly impacted the course of Tibetan medicine. Tibetan medicine practitioners and practices have suffered persecution and censorship, particularly during the Cultural Revolution. Yet, compared with many of Tibet's religious and cultural institutions, Tibetan medicine is thought to have emerged from the ravages of the 1950s, '60s, and '70s relatively intact. Particularly since reforms began in the late 1970s in China, the PRC government has sanctioned the study, clinical practice, and research-oriented advancement of Tibetan medicine. In addition to Chinese governmental support, today Tibetan medicine is also supported by a variety of non-governmental organisations (NGOs).

- *Sowa rigpa*, Tibet's 'science of healing', bears comparison to Traditional Chinese Medicine (TCM), as well as to Indian Ayurveda, ancient Greek, Persian and Central Asian medicine, although it is not reducible to a 'branch' or 'subset' of either. In the context of the PRC, this cultural and medical system has been aligned more with 'science' than with 'religion' by the Chinese state, which has helped legitimate state support for Tibetan medicine. Yet this support has had both positive and negative impacts on Tibetan medical practitioners, clinical practice, education and the production of Tibetan medicines themselves.

- Contemporary Tibetan medical practitioners are facing the challenges of finding new ways to keep younger generations engaged in, devoted to and gainfully employed by Tibetan medical practice. They are also dealing with the difficulties and possibilities inherent in shifts toward the institutionalisation of Tibetan medical education, in state and/or NGO-funded schools, and away from private, lineage-based master-apprentice transmission of medical knowledge.

- Contemporary Tibetan doctors are also dealing with the relationship between Tibetan medicine and biomedicine. Key to this interaction are questions about how to provide the best possible health care for Tibetan communities, as well as training and clinical opportunities for young Tibetan doctors, while not losing what is unique about Tibetan medicine in an attempt to 'integrate' these two systems of medical knowledge. This includes topics such as the relationship between each system's pharmacopoeia, treatment regimes and clinical practice, as well as larger issues such as how 'health' or 'illness' is defined and on what basis diagnosis is made.

- Over the last decades, there has been a shift away from the making of medicines by *amchi*, or Tibetan doctors, themselves, to the larger-scale production of medicines in factories. Tibetan medicines are becoming commercialised, and factories are facing government and international pressures to standardise production and patent Tibetan formulas. This shift in how medicines are produced and prescribed bears directly on the efficacy of the medicines themselves, as well as patients' and doctors' perceptions of the power and quality of Tibetan medical healing practices.

- The pressures to standardise and commercialise Tibetan pharmaceuticals also relate to the future of Tibet's specific ecology and the stresses placed on it by the trade in medicinal plants, in particular. Some efforts at conserving the rare and endangered species on which Tibetan medicine depends and cultivating a variety of medicinal plants has begun within Tibetan areas of the PRC. However, such endeavours are still at an early stage.

- Tibetan medical institutions, both within and outside the PRC, are today engaged in a variety of clinical research projects, often using biomedical methods such as those of the Randomised Controlled Trial as a basis for research design and measurements of 'success.' These activities create opportunities for Tibetan medicines to be available to patients around the world, but they also raise fundamental issues such as how to translate between medical systems, as well as concerns over Intellectual Property Rights (IPR) and questions about what the impacts of such research will be on the future availability of Tibetan medicine to Tibetan communities, both within and outside the PRC.

- The hybrid approach of practising both types of medicine in the same settings by the same doctor provides, in principle, the possibility that the patient can benefit from 'the best of both worlds'. This pragmatic approach, though, obviously requires the full recognition of and support for traditional Tibetan medicine. Without such special support, any traditional approach will always be confronted by the internationalised pressure of modern biomedicine, and ultimately degraded to the status of a 'little sibling', which will then only be administered from time in an opportunistic manner.

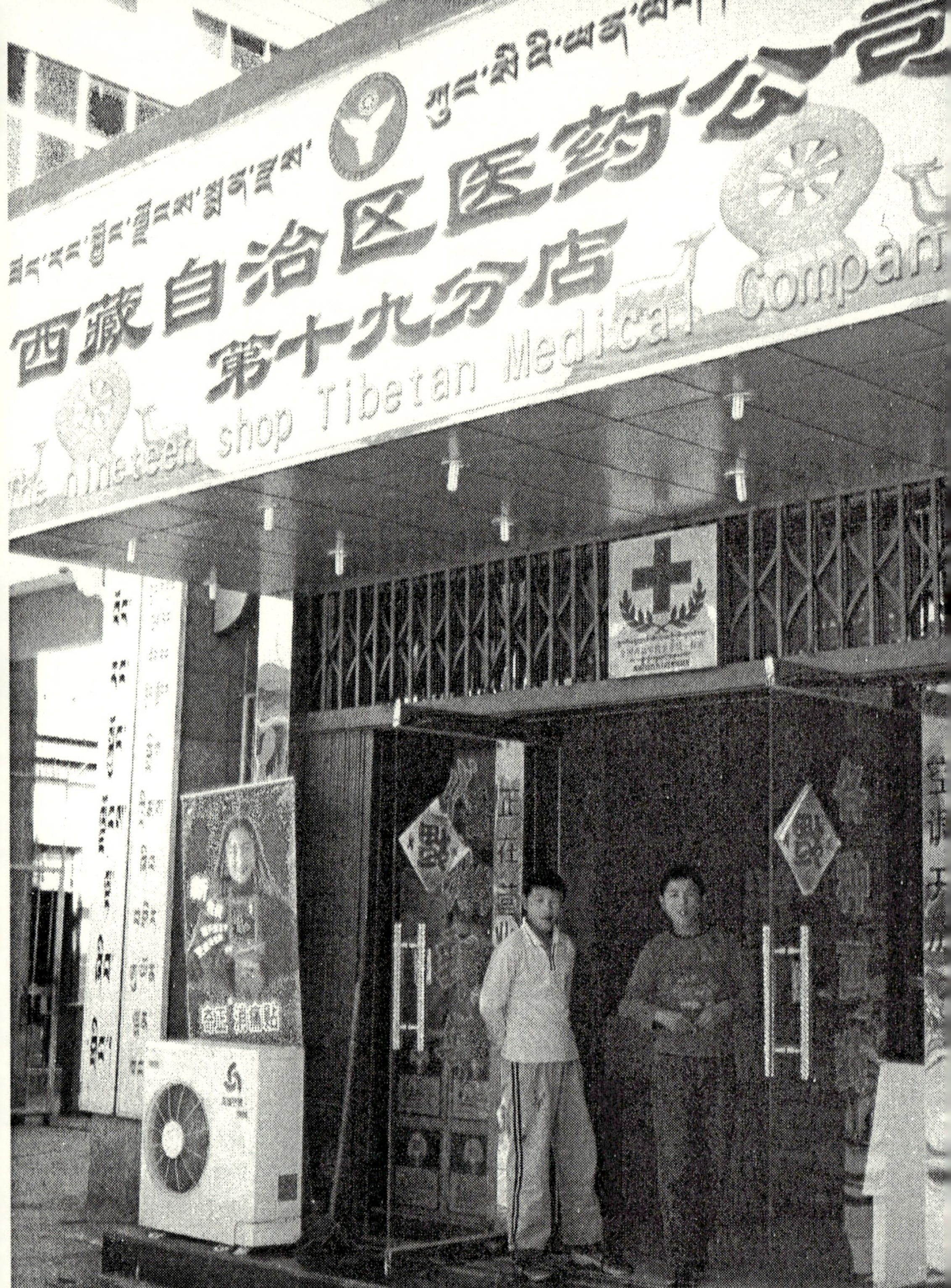

Tibetan medicine store on Yuthog Lam, Lhasa
© TIN

Introduction

This TIN book, the second in a series on health and health care in Tibet, examines the relationship between Tibetan medicine and contemporary Tibetan society. It attempts to provide the general public and those who know Tibet well with an understanding of the ways that Tibetan medical practice has changed in Tibet since 1959, but with emphasis on the period from the early 1980s to the present, and with particular emphasis on the TAR and institutes of Tibetan medicine in Lhasa. We recognise that to generalise about the vast landscapes and diverse communities that make up the Tibetan areas of the PRC is difficult, but we believe that a general overview of the trends to do with Tibetan medicine in these areas is still worthwhile. We aim to balance discussions of clinical practice and access to Tibetan medicine in urban and rural Tibetan communities with discussions of Tibetan medical education. We will also discuss the roles of non-governmental organisations (NGOs), foreign researchers, exile Tibetan communities and the Chinese state in the perpetuation of and challenges facing Tibetan medicine today. Although the book begins with a brief introduction to the history, pharmacology, diagnosis and treatment methods of this medical tradition, as well as a sketch of the relationship between medicine and religious philosophy and practice, this is not the primary focus of this book. Rather, we are concerned with the perpetuation of Tibetan medicine in today's Tibet, as well as its future prospects as a science, healing art, an affordable and available component of the health care systems at work in Tibet, and an indicator of cultural, linguistic, and religious survival.

This story of Tibetan medicine today is told against the backdrop of the expanding global marketplace for 'alternative' medicines and therapies, from the fame and funding associated with this trend, to the concrete harm and benefit that this demand for non-western or non-biomedical approaches to health and healing can have on the societies and ecologies from which these therapies are derived. In addition, the specific circumstances of Tibetan medicine in contemporary Tibet illustrate another more global theme: the propensity for governments and non-governmental organisations to simultaneously promote scientific, medical, and technological advancement – one definition of 'development' – and to capitalise on the traditions of 'minority' groups. Although there can be positive outcomes from such interactions, one result of this dynamic – the tug-of-war between tradition and modernity – can be the appropriation and commodification of knowledge systems, practices and natural resources, and the wresting of control and confidence over these practices from their true inheritors. Although the particular story of Tibetan medicine in contemporary Tibet, and in the People's Republic of China, is less grim than other aspects of Tibet's recent political and cultural history, it is a tale of contradiction, dramatic change and an uncertain future.

This book examines the social, political, and economic issues that are impacting the use, availability and production of Tibetan medicine, as well as the cultural identity associated with Tibetan medicine in contemporary Tibet. The book begins by sketching the history of Tibetan medicine, with particular reference to its founding medical institutions in historical Tibet, and how these institutions have changed since the 1950s. It also examines the relationship between religious and medical instruction and practice. Chapter Two follows from this introduction to explore Tibetan medical education in a modern context, with particular attention to the changes in how such knowledge is transmitted from one generation to another and the formation of new kinds of schools and training programmes for Tibetan medicine, many of them funded by foreign NGOs. Chapter Three is a study of Tibetan pharmaceuticals and connections between availability, profit and efficacy. It focuses on the production and commercialisation of Tibetan medicines, including the changing availability of medicinal plants and other *materia medica*, the growth of the Tibetan medical industry in the TAR and other parts of China, the impact of government relations on production techniques and the demand for and limitations of selling Tibetan remedies internationally. While Chapter Two addresses the making of a Tibetan physician, and Chapter Three addresses the making of Tibetan medicines, Chapter Four examines contemporary clinical practice in a variety of settings, from private homes and clinics to government hospitals. This chapter also discusses in more detail the relationship between 'Western' biomedicine and Tibetan medicine. Here, we pay attention to the increasing influence of biomedical methods, treatments, and technologies within the context of Tibetan medical practice. Chinese government and foreign NGO interventions into, and attempts to integrate, these two medical systems through public health policy, health training and development programmes, and medical research are also considered. This book concludes with some observations on the place of 'traditional' Tibetan medicine in this 'modern' world, and the circumstances under which it exists in the People's Republic of China (PRC) today.

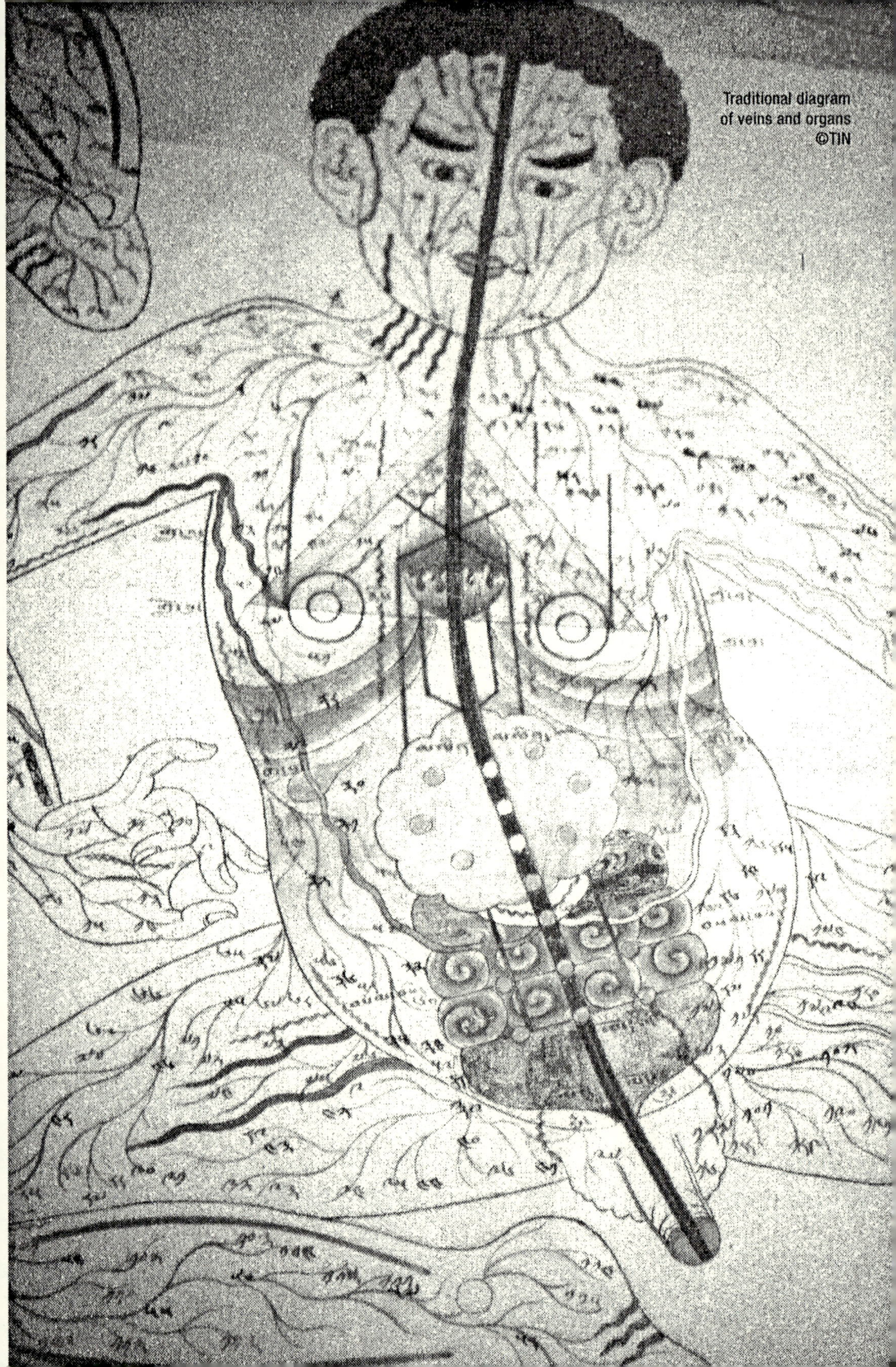

Traditional diagram
of veins and organs
©TIN

Chapter One

Tibetan Medicine:
Principles, Past and Present

Tibetan medicine has been practiced since at least the seventh century. However, the Chinese annexation of Tibet in the 1950s and the subsequent Tibetan diaspora have greatly impacted the course of Tibetan medicine. Tibetans-in-exile have established institutions for medical training in India, the foremost among which are the Tibetan Medical and Astrological Institute (TMAI), also known as the Men-tsee-khang, in Dharamsala, and Chagpori Medical Institute in Darjeeling. Likewise, the Chinese government has sanctioned the study and advancement of Tibetan medicine in the Tibet Autonomous Region (TAR) and parts of Qinghai, Sichuan, Gansu and Yunnan Provinces, areas that Tibetans know as Kham and Amdo.

This has been true particularly since reform movements began from 1978 – a move that can be interpreted as their efforts to incorporate Tibetan cultural forms into China's nationalist project. Furthermore, Tibetan medicine is experiencing a renaissance in other parts of South and Central Asia, particularly in Mongolia and parts of the former Soviet Union. Today, whether in exile or in Tibet, contemporary Tibetan medical practitioners are confronting new health risks, including AIDS, for which the classical medical curriculum has not necessarily prepared them. They are also facing the challenges of transitioning from what was historically a lineage-based practice into a profession, and of finding new ways to keep younger generations engaged in and devoted to Tibetan medical practice. Tibetan medical institutions, both within the PRC and in exile, are also engaged in research into the treatment of chronic diseases such as cancer, hepatitis, and diabetes, thus attempting to prove the efficacy of their system in western scientific terms. And Tibetan medicines themselves are becoming commercialised, and factories are facing pressures to standardise and patent Tibetan formulas.

But before exploring these changes and challenges in more depth, particularly in reference to life inside Tibet, we provide a brief overview of the history, epistemology, pharmacology, and treatment methods of Tibetan medicine in order to place these changes in context. We hope that, from this basis, readers may not only come to understand something of the vast changes that are occurring within Tibetan medicine – as it interacts with biomedicine, nationalist agendas and big business, for instance – but that they are also able to more fully appreciate the science and art of the Tibetan system of healing in its own right.

Tibetan Medicine: Basic Principles and Practices[1]

To begin, it is important to remember that not only Tibetan medical history but also Tibetan conceptions of illness and disease are integrally linked to Buddhism and Buddhist philosophy, as well as to Bön, the title generally given to the pre-Buddhist religious traditions of Tibet.

What is Bön Medicine?

Generally speaking, Bön is the name given to the diversity of ritual practices and worldviews that comprise the 'pre-Buddhist' religion(s) of Tibet. A 6th century BC figure known as Shenrab Miboche is said to be the founder of The Nine Ways of Bön – or the Bön religion. Shenrab Miboche and Bön are also associated with the ancient Tibetan kingdom of Shang Shung (present-day Ngari Prefecture, TAR).

Among the works attributed to Shenrab Miboche is the *Sorig Bumshi*, a corpus of medical and medico-religious teachings that parallel the *Gyushi*, the Four Medical Tantras in Tibetan Buddhist tradition. Practitioners and some scholars of Bön argue that this text was added to and rewritten from the 6th century BC through the 8th century AD, and that it not only predates the Buddhist *gyushi*, but that it is also one of the oldest medical texts in the world. The *bumshi* relates a system of healing connected to the four elements, as illustrated by the following quotation attributed to Shenrab Miboche: *Our state of health as well as diseases are influenced by the four elements. Similarly, the medications prepared from plants and minerals are also under the influence of these elements* (Kletter and Kriechbaum 2001).

Today, the distinctions between Tibetan Buddhism and Bön, as well as between Buddhist and Bön *sowa rigpa* are topics of scholarly and practical debate, often wrapped up in political agendas and identity politics. Some say that the medical systems are distinct, while others contest that they are quite similar, particularly at this point in history; some argue that Bön religious and medical practices are the more 'authentically' Tibetan, since the practices are older and pre-date Buddhist influence. Regardless of this, it can be said with confidence that identifying oneself as practicing or studying Bön medicine is a way of asserting a specific social identity: Bön had not been officially recognised by the Tibetan state before 1959 – and had sometimes come under attack – and was not officially recognised by the Tibetan government-in-exile as one of the official religious schools of Tibet until the 1990s. Today, practitioners of *sowa rigpa* who identify themselves as Bönpo (followers of Bön), exist throughout the TAR and other Tibetan areas of the PRC. Some practice as spirit mediums and oracles (*lhapa* or *lhamo*), while others practice medicine in ways that are virtually indistinguishable to the non-specialist from their Buddhist counterparts.

---

1 The work of many scholars informs this brief synopsis of Tibetan medical theory. Chief among these sources are the works of Clark, Dhonden, Dummer, Fenton, and Meyer, as well as *The Fundamentals of Tibetan Medicine* and the series *Tibetan Medicine*, both published by the Men-tsee-Khang in Dharamsala, India (full citations in bibliography).

Scholars and practitioners of *sowa rigpa* – literally the Tibetan 'science of healing' – recognise, appreciate, and debate the historical origins of their practice. Yet at a deeper level, the inspired centre of Tibetan medicine is attributed to the teaching of the Master of Remedies, popularly known as the Medicine Buddha (*Sangye Menla;* Skt. *Bhaishajya Guru*). Unlike western biomedical practice, which views the body as a physiological composite, Tibetan medicine views illness, suffering, and healing as a fully embodied experience – located not only in physical body but also in mind and spirit. In Tibetan medical epistemology, healing and illness are fundamentally connected to the basic tenets of Buddhism: that suffering – and, as such, illness – arises from desire, anger and ignorance, and that the cessation of suffering is possible by following the Buddha's path. The *Gyushi* or Four Medical Tantras form the core of Tibetan medical curriculum. But these volumes are not only – or not simply – medical textbooks. They contain prayers and ritual instruction as well as treatises on pharmacology and epidemiology, diagnosis and treatment. Similarly, the Kangyur and Tengyur, the complete sutras of the Buddha and their commentaries, respectively, also include medical exegesis.

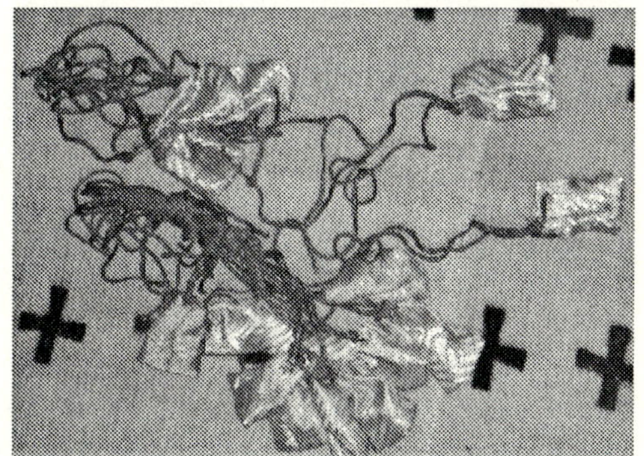

Like ancient Greek medicine as well as Ayurveda (the traditional Indian medicine system), Tibetan medicine has come to be classified as a 'humoral' practice. In the specific context of Tibetan medicine, this basically means a system of healing based on the balance of specific elements; the word often translated as 'humour' in Tibetan, *nyepa*, is actually the same word for 'illness' and 'fault'. The Three Humours (*nyepa sum*) in Tibetan medicine are *loong, tripa*, and *bekhen*, which are roughly translated as wind, bile, and phlegm; they correspond to Ayurveda's divisions of *vatta, pitta*, and *kapha*. Yet the distinctions between and within the humours are different in *sowa rigpa* and Ayurveda. And, unlike Ayurveda, this state of health also depends on a balance of the Five Elements (*chung wa nga*): earth (*sa*), water (*chu*), fire (*me*), air (*loong*), and space (*nam kha*). The three humours are

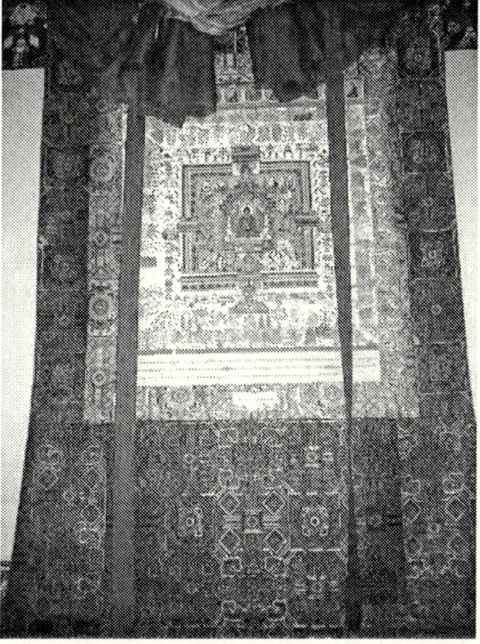

Top: Protection cords ('sung') with medicine   © TIN
Above: Thanka of Sangye Menla   ©TIN

associated with these five cosmo-physical elements: the wind element is associated with *loong*, fire with *tripa*, and the combination of earth and water with *bekhen*. Within *sowa rigpa*, then, health is a state of balance: moments when the three humours and the five elements are maintained in a state of equilibrium within an individual. Treatment involves balancing the three humours. In this sense, Tibetan medicine is an allopathic medical system, in that balance is restored and treatment prescribed by giving a patient medicine or other therapies that correspond with the humours opposite those that are out of balance.[2] An imbalance that Tibetan medicine determines as 'hot' is treated with 'cold' remedies, and vice versa. Homeopathic medicine, in contrast, treats an illness with likeness as opposed to difference, relying on derivatives of the same substance that creates a particular illness.

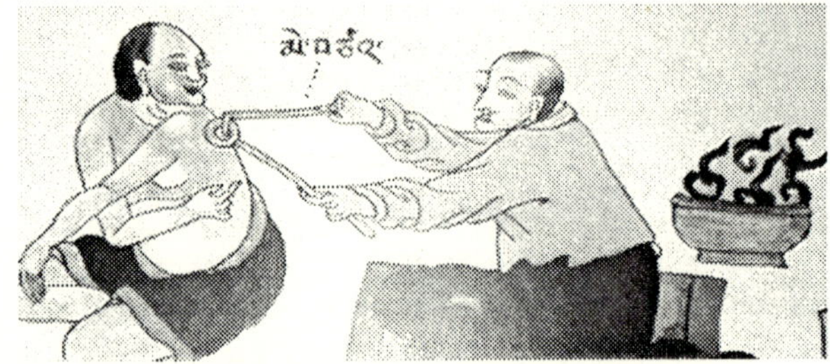
Cupping, one of the traditional therapy methods ©TIN

So, while Tibetan medicine and western biomedicine can both be considered as allopathic systems, in the strict sense of the term, these two methods of healing are different in the way they conceive of disease. Biomedicine tends to classify diseases, define symptoms, and then treat according to these symptoms. Tibetan medicine does not treat diseases *per se*, but rather addresses particular imbalances within a given treatment. However, this is not to say that Tibetan medicine does not give names to specific disorders. When one observes Tibetan medicine being practiced clinically, or when one reads Tibetan medical texts, specific disorders are classified according to which humour, or combination of humours, is the dominant one causing this state of 'imbalance' in a patient. *Sowa rigpa* distinguishes between primary and secondary causes of illness at the level of medical philosophy, as well as at the level of clinical practice. Within the Tibetan medical worldview, the primary cause of illness or imbalance is articulated as *ma rigpa*, ignorance, and directly links this medical system with Tibetan Buddhism's theory of *duk sum*, or the Three Poisons: attachment, hatred and delusion. Within this theory of the primary cause of illness, each of the three humours links up with one of the three poisons that, in Buddhist doctrine, cause the perpetuation of suffering and *samsara*, cyclic existence. *Loong* corresponds to attachment and desire, *tripa* is related to hatred and *bekhen* relates to delusion and narrow mindedness. Beyond this, the secondary causes of illness stem from psychic and physiological imbalances of the three humours and five elements, and are rooted in diet, inadequate behaviour, the actions of evil spirits and the *karma* of past lives.

According to Tibetan medical texts and the teachings of the Medicine Buddha, there are 84,000 different kinds of afflictive emotions, including desire, hatred, and delusion, that produce 84,000 different kinds of disorders. These disorders are further condensed into 404 main humoral imbalances, which are in turn treated by Tibetan medicines and therapies, from herbal pills to spiritual practices. These 404 main humoral imbalances

---

2 What we know as 'Western' medicine or biomedicine is also an allopathic system. 'Allopathy' is defined as the treatment of disease by inducing an opposite condition, and is the opposite of homeopathy.

play out in the clinical context through the ways treatment regimes are prioritised. For instance, if a person is diagnosed with both a serious *loong* disorder and more mild *tripa*-related disorder, the physician might choose to first treat the *tripa* disorder and, once the patient's overall strength is a bit better, treat the more serious *loong* imbalance.

Listed below are the humours and their natures.

- ***Loong*** is both hot and cold in nature. It is rough, light, cold, subtle, and moist. There are five different kinds of *loong*: the life-sustaining *loong* governs the brain, senses and intellect; the ascending *loong* bears on the chest, speech and memory; the all-pervading *loong* corresponds to the heart and movement; the fire-accompanying *loong* is connected to the stomach and digestion; and the downward-cleansing *loong* corresponds to the pelvis and excretions, binding a body to the earth.

- ***Tripa*** is hot in nature. It is described as oily, sharp, hot, light, fetid, purgative and moist. There are five different kinds of *tripa*: digestive *tripa* relates to the stomach and gastro-intestinal function; the accompanying *tripa* is connected with the heart, mental discretion, anger and ambition; colour regulating *tripa* corresponds to the liver and blood; sight giving *tripa* link to the eyes; and complexion clearing *tripa* relates to the skin.

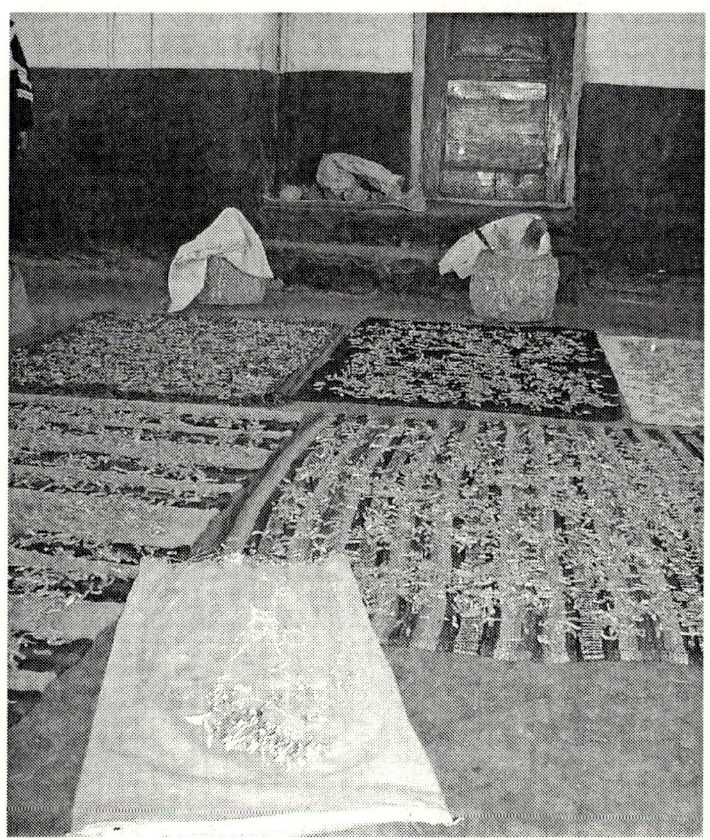

Drying ingredients   ©TIN

• **Bekhen** is cold in nature. It is described as oily, cool, heavy, blunt, smooth, firm and sticky. There are five kinds of *bekhen*: supportive *bekhen* corresponds to the chest; decomposing *bekhen* relates to the stomach; experiencing *bekhen* links to the

Humours, elements and soma

Humours (nyepa sum)		Associated elements (chung wa nga)	Links to the 'Three poisons' (druk sum)	Nature of humours		Humours' sub-categories	Psycho-physiological links
Tibetan	English			hot/cold	qualities		
loong	wind	wind/air *(loong)*	attachment + desire	hot & cold	rough, light, cold, subtle, moist	life-sustaining *loong*	brain, senses, intellect
						ascending *loong*	chest, speech, memory
						all-pervading *loong*	heart, movement
						fire-accompanying *loong*	stomach, digestion
						downward-cleansing *loong*	pelvis, excretions
tripa	bile	fire *(me)*	hatred	hot	oily, sharp, hot, light, fetid, purgative, moist	digestive *tripa*	stomach, gastro-intestinal function
						accompanying *tripa*	heart, mental discretion, anger and ambition
						colour regulating *tripa*	liver, blood
						sight giving *tripa*	eyes
						complexion clearing *tripa*	skin
bekhen	phlegm	earth + water *(sa + chu)*	delusion/ narrow mindedness	cold	oily, cool, heavy, blunt, smooth, firm and sticky	supportive *bekhen*	chest
						decomposing *bekhen*	stomach
						experiencing *bekhen*	tongue
						satisfying *bekhen*	head, level of sensitivity of the five senses
						connective *bekhen*	joints
(no correspondence)		space *(nam kha)*					

tongue; satisfying *bekhen* links to the head and level of sensitivity of the five senses increase in sensitivity; finally, connective *bekhen* resides in the joints.

The Seven Bodily Constituents (*lu sung duen*), the Six Tastes (*ro druk*), and the three post-digestive tastes, as well as the eight potentialities of medicinal ingredients, are also a part of the puzzle of the sentient body – in sickness and in health. These seven bodily constituents are nutritional essence, blood, muscle tissue, fatty tissue, bone, bone marrow, and regenerative essences/reproductive fluids. The six tastes are: sweet, sour, salty, bitter, hot, and astringent, while the three post-digestive tastes are sweet, acid and bitter. The eight potentialities of medicinal drugs are heavy, light, unctuous, pungent, cold, warm, blunted, and incisive. Like the three humours, the seven bodily constituents and the six tastes are also connected to the five elements. This balance of humours, tastes, constituents and elements creates a web of meaning and experience, within which a patient's state of being is considered and treated. For example, subdivisions of the six tastes relate to sensory perception and to the ability of Tibetan doctors to feel and classify medicines, as well as to diagnose imbalances; they are used in combination to restore balance in the patient, and also relate to *sowa rigpa*'s complex pharmacology.

The Tibetan medical system is described and studied using visual aids, particularly those from the 'Illustrated Trees of Medicine', a series of *thangka*, or traditional Tibetan scroll

The 'Illustrated Tree of Medicine' (simplified)				
3 Roots	**9 Trunks**	**42 Branches**	**224 Leaves, 2 flowers, 3 fruits**	
'Definition of the body'	healthy body	humoral balance	flowers	freedom from disease
				long life
		physical constituents	fruits	religious practice
				wealth
		excretions		happiness
	imbalanced/unhealthy body	causes and conditions giving rise to illness	88 leaves	
		ways illness enter the body		
		location of illness		
		times illness arises		
		fatal effects of illness		
'Diagnosis root'	visual observation of the patient	8 branches	38 leaves	
	pulse analysis			
	questions to the patient			
'Healing root'	foods	27 branches	98 leaves	
	behaviours			
	medicines			
	accessory therapies			

paintings. In these illustrations, we come to see Tibetan medicine as a system of three roots from which grow nine trunks and on which there are 42 branches, 224 leaves, as well as two flowers and three fruits. The first of the three roots is called 'Definition of the Body'. It is further divided into two trunks, one representing the healthy body and the second representing the unbalanced or unhealthy body. The branches of the healthy body trunk discuss things such as humoral balance, physical constituents and excretions, as well as the two flowers – freedom from disease and long life – and the three fruits – religious practice, wealth and happiness. The diseased body trunk, on the other hand, discusses the causes and conditions giving rise to illness as well as the ways illness enters the body, the locations of illness, the times illnesses arise, and the fatal effects of illness. The second of these three roots is the 'Diagnosis Root', which is comprised of three trunks, eight branches, and 38 leaves. These three trunks describe visual observation of the patient, including examination of the patient's tongue and urine; pulse analysis; and questioning the patient, each in relation to the balance of the three humours within a given individual. The third and final root is the 'Healing Root', which includes four trunks, 27 branches, and 98 leaves. The four trunks describe foods, behaviours, medicines and accessory therapies, such as moxibustion, that are used to treat illnesses.

As the trees describe, Tibetan medical diagnosis is performed primarily through pulse and urine analysis, examining the tongue of the patient and listening to the patient's history. It is fair to say that diagnosis is a complex science and art. As in traditional Chinese medicine, pulse diagnosis also takes years of practice to master. Pulses are felt for their speed, quality and other characteristics. There are twelve organ pulses, felt under six fingers on three different levels. There are many different kinds of pulses: constitutional, seasonal, lifespan, pregnancy, vital and vessel organs. Urine analysis is done to examine the urine for colour, taste and consistency, while examination of the patient's tongue reveals another level of information about the patient's humoral state. Patient history includes asking questions about diet, behaviour, lifestyle, the person's emotional and mental state, physical problems and dreams.

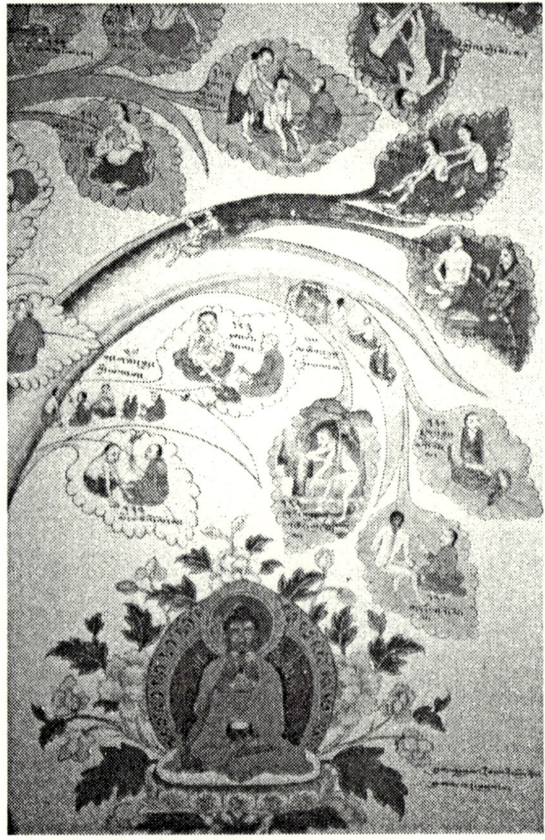

The Tree of Medicine, detail   ©TIN

Once a diagnosis is made, a Tibetan doctor, called an *amchi* or *menpa* in Tibetan, might prescribe any number of treatments, first among which are pills or powders, to be chewed and swallowed with hot water. Tibetan medicines are primarily herbal-based, although many medicines also include minerals, precious and semi-precious stones, and some animal products. There is no medicine that is comprised of a single plant or other ingredient. It is most common to have at least six different ingredients in a given medicine. Other methods of treatment include moxibustion, bloodletting, cupping, herbal baths, massage, golden needle acupuncture (*ser khab*), herbal stick therapy, incense, the wearing of protective amulets, the ingesting of ritual blessing pills, called *chinlab* or *mani rilbu*, and a variety of healing rituals, which, depending on context, are either performed by a ritual specialist such as a Buddhist priest or an oracle, or by an *amchi*. Other forms of treatment include restrictions on diet and behaviour. Historically, most Tibetan doctors produced their own medicines. However, as we shall explore in more detail in Chapter Three, a shift away from the making of medicines by *amchi* themselves, to the larger-scale production of medicines in factories has been occurring within and outside the PRC. This is particularly true of contemporary Tibet, and bears directly on the efficacy of the medicines themselves, as well as patients' and doctors' perceptions of the power and quality of *sowa rigpa* healing practices.

Let us now turn from Tibetan medical principles to an examination of its history, as a means of further establishing a foundation from which to understand the changes occurring within Tibetan medicine today.

A Brief History of Tibetan Medicine[3]

It is difficult to separate the evolutions of Tibet's science of healing from the rise and dissemination of Buddhism from India across the Tibetan Plateau. Although external influences on Tibetan medical practice range from China to Byzantium, from India to the Mongolian steppe, and although Tibetan medicine as a system of healing incorporates much pre-Buddhist indigenous knowledge and practices, the creation of a corpus of Tibetan medical texts and the systematic development of Tibetan medical logic is integrally tied to the history of Buddhism in Tibet. However, it is important to remember Buddhism's position as the official state religion during the 'imperial' or 'dynastic' Tibetan age (634-842 AD).[4] Likewise, we should be mindful of the ways that this historical fact has influenced the development not only of Tibetan medical practice, but also of historical memory. In other words: *One should approach Tibetan medical history with an understanding that the lines between myth and historical fact are often blurred, that Buddhist doctrine incorporated, converted and was contested by pre-Buddhist healing practices, and that the Tibetan language sources that trace this history were often*

---

3 Many scholars' works have informed, and helped to structure, this condensed history of Tibetan medicine. In particular, we have drawn on the works of Clifford, Dhonden, Dummer, Gerke, Gyatso, McKay, Meyer, Rechung, Samuel, and Unkrig (full citations in bibliography).
4 The period of Tibet's early medieval history known by turns as the 'imperial' or 'dynastic' age, began in the seventh century, with the rise to power of the Tsenpo lineage of kings in the Yarlung Valley east of present-day Lhasa, and lasted until the mid-ninth century. Before this time, what we know today as Central and Eastern Tibet were ruled by rival chiefs.

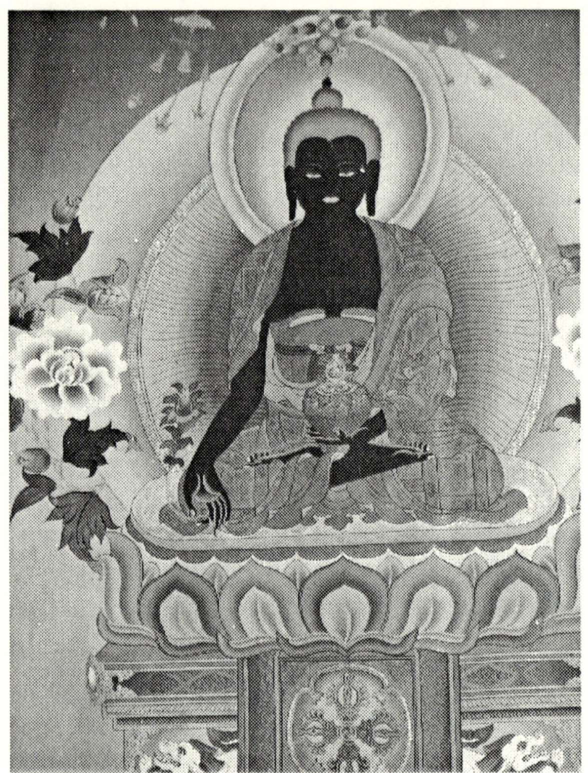

Sangye Menla   ©TIN

compiled centuries after the events to which they refer; sometimes it is impossible to distinguish history from legend. (Kapstein 2000: 23)

That being said, two specific periods in early Tibetan history emerge in the development of sowa rigpa: that of the first (*nga dar*) and second (*chi dar*) dissemination of Buddhism in Tibet. From the 7th through the 9th centuries, the Tibetan empire flourished. This period is marked by the development of a Tibetan script, which made possible the translation of Sanskrit, Chinese and other bodies of literature and scientific knowledge into Tibetan language. Manuscripts that comprise part of the Dunhuang (Tun-huang) cave collections corroborate many of these early Chinese and Indian influences. These caves, located in present-day Xinjiang Province (Chinese Turkestan), at the far eastern edge of the Taklamakan Desert, held ancient archives that included many thousands of Tibetan volumes on history, medicine, religion, astrology, and other topics.[5] During this first dissemination of Buddhism in Tibet, the influences on indigenous medical practices are said to have come primarily from Greek, Chinese, and Sanskritic sources. Like other imperial eras, this period was a formative stage for Tibetan society, politics, economics and culture, including Tibetan medicine.

Chief among these formative moments in Tibetan history were the courts of two Tibetan kings: Songtsen Gampo (617 – 649/650 AD) and Trisong Detsen (742 – 797 AD). During the reign of Songtsen Gampo, physicians of Greek, Indian and Chinese origin were invited to the Tibetan court, bringing with them both literary sources and medical texts, as well as much orally transmitted medical knowledge. Although only the Greek physician was said to have stayed on in Tibet as court physician, these different schools of medicine had a profound influence on the development of Tibetan medical practice.

---

5 Snellgrove and Richardson describe, "[In the Tun-huang caves] *there had survived for ten centuries and more collections of ancient manuscripts, hermetically sealed from the ravages of the outside world. The collections, which were subsequently brought to Europe* [after being discovered by scholar-explorers Sir Aurel Stein and Professor Paul Pelliot], *were divided between libraries in London (the India Office Library) and Paris (Bibliothèque Nationale). Only a small part of the material is Tibetan, most of which consists of Buddhist texts, but there are some non-Buddhist records, one of which summarizes events of the royal court and the principal affairs of state, while others contain rather more literary and poetic versions of those occurrences and also legends relating to the mythical origins of the country*" (1995: 76-77).

In addition, two of Songtsen Gampo's wives, one of Nepali noble origin and the other a Chinese Tang Dynasty princess, carried with them to Tibet many medical and astrological texts, some of which were subsequently brought into the fold of *sowa rigpa*. Incidentally, this relationship between the Tibetan imperial court and the Tang emperors was crucial, not only in the history of Tibetan medicine but also in the larger geo-political context of the relationship between Chinese and Tibetan cultures, worldviews and military powers.

King Trisong Detsen was said to have nine court physicians who hailed from India, Kashmir, China, Iran, East Turkestan and Nepal, as well as areas on the margins of the Tibetan Empire, such as Dolpo in present-day Nepal. During this time, medical exchange between

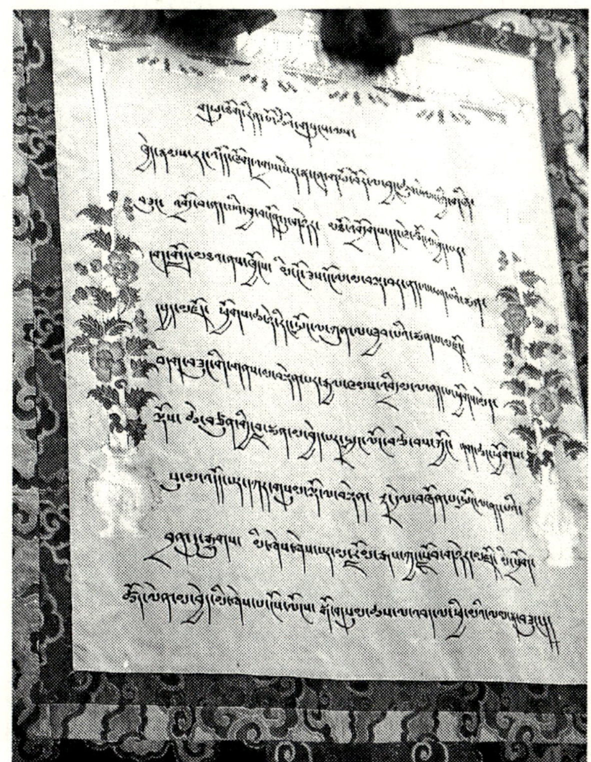

Edict of Yutok Yonten Gompo   ©TIN

traditions flourished, and influenced the further development of *sowa rigpa*. One of the most influential court physicians during this period was Yuthog Yonten Gompo the Elder. This Tibetan physician is credited with founding a new medical school and one of the most influential medical lineages in Tibetan history. Yuthog Yonten Gompo the Elder was also said to have studied Ayurveda at Nalanda, the famous institution of higher learning in what is today North India, and to have lived for 125 years.

The later propagation of Buddhism in Tibet marked the consolidation of earlier medical texts and the introduction of new works, primarily of Indic origin. It also marked the large-scale development of Tibetan monastic institutions, many of which also incorporated medical education and practice. During this time, the *Gyushi* or the *Four Medical Tantra* – books that comprise key *sowa rigpa* medical teachings – were edited and added to, resulting in the form they still retain today: four volumes, comprising 159 chapters. Chief among the influences on *sowa rigpa* during this later propagation was Yuthog Yonten Gompo the Younger (1112 – 1203 AD). Yuthog Yonten Gompo the Younger is generally acknowledged to have edited and revised the works comprising the *Gyushi*, as well as to have written commentaries on many sections. In addition to his work on the *Gyushi*, Yuthog the Younger also authored about 20 other medical works, including the first text that presented a history of Tibetan medicine. However, the origins of the *Gyushi* remain a topic of scholarly debate: some say that although the text shows influence from many sources, it is a decidedly Tibetan work; some insist it is a translation of an Indian work, the Astangahridayasamhita by Vagbhata; others still fall somewhere in between. Significantly, the master translator Rinchen Zangpo (958-1055 AD) translated this Sanskrit text into Tibetan, and is also said to have devoted much of his scholarly attention to medical topics. Beyond this scholarly debate, many Tibetans consider the Gyushi a terma or a treasure text said to be revealed at an auspicious time; terma texts often serve to legitimate the lineage and spiritual authenticity of a particular set of ideas, teachings and practices.

What is in the *Gyushi?*

The more complete title of the *Gyushi* is *A Treatise of Secret Oral Transmission of the Nectar of Medical Knowledge*. The *Gyushi* contains 156 chapters, 5900 verses, which deal with the eight branches of medicine: the body, including embryology, anatomy, physiology, pathology, pharmacology, etc., as well as paediatrics, gynaecology, disorders caused by evil spirits, wounds inflicted by trauma, toxicology, rejuvenation and aphrodisiacs. The four volumes are broken down as follows:

1 – The Root Tantra (*Tsa gyu*) is a summary of all the Tibetan medical teachings
2 – The Explanatory Tantra (*Shey gyu*) is a detailed account of embryology, physiology, etc.
3 – The Oral Instruction Tantra (*Men ngag gyu*) is a description of specific illnesses and treatments.
4 – The Last Tantra (*Chima gyu*) details pulse and urine diagnosis, pacification of disease, evacuation and accessory therapies. It is the most general of the Four Tantra.

With the exception of the Oral Instruction Tantra, all the texts were memorised over a period of approximately five years, according to traditional Tibetan medical education systems. The Oral Instruction Tantra is usually not memorised because it contains 92 chapters and is very long; instead, sections of this text are memorised. Today, students of Tibetan medicine must still memorise significant parts of the Gyushi, though the scope of, and emphasis placed on, this memorisation has changed. See Chapter Two for more details.

The *Gyushi* often reads like religious instruction, which shows the further interrelation between Tibetan Buddhism and Tibetan medicine, particularly at the level of textual knowledge. Consider the following passage, taken from a translation of the Explanatory Tantra of the *Gyushi*:

"With respect to the prerequisites, the doctor should be intelligent, altruistic, adhering to his words of honour, knowledgeable in practice, diligent and well-versed in social mores...The six factors to be kept in [the] mind [of the physician] are the preceptor, his teaching, the medical treatises, one's fellow students, the patient and the latter's bodily constituents. Considering the preceptor as the Buddha, his teachings as the speech of the rishi, the medical treatises as the Oral Instruction Lineage, one's fellow students as friends and relatives, patients as one's children and their bodily constituents as one's pet...one should maintain the apprehension of the Medicine Holder of Knowledge as an out-bound protector and his medical instruments as the latter's instruments...Medicine is to be understood in a threefold way – as precious gems, as nectar and as offering substances. One should perceive it as a wish-fulfilling gem accomplishing one's needs and desires. It should also be perceived as a nectar that dispels diseases and, as the primary offering substance of a vidhayadhara, or Knowledge Holder...These precious medicines should be sought out and retained...and should be well compounded and consecrated as nectar. The physician should think of himself as the 'King of Aquamarine Light', consider the medicine container as a begging bowl filled with nectar and the visualised retinue of rishis around him as chanting auspiciously." (Clark 1995: 224-225)

From both a sociological and an historical perspective, Tibetan medical practice has been structured around lineage-based master-apprentice relationships. Here, lineage or *gyu* refers to both modes of knowledge transmission from teacher to disciple, usually in a monastic context, or through patrilineal descent, often from father to son or uncle to nephew. In this light, this is why figures like Yuthog Yongen Gompo the Elder and the Younger are so pivotal in the history of Tibetan medicine, not only because of their vast clinical and scholarly knowledge, but also because they lent legitimacy, through lineage, to future generations of *amchi*, practitioners of Tibetan medicine. As we shall explore in more detail in Chapter Two, the role of lineage in the perpetuation of Tibetan medicine remains an important – yet changing – element of Tibetan medical practice today. From the 15th to the 17th centuries, two main schools of Tibetan medicine developed under different master lineage holders: the Northern School (*chang lug*) and the Southern School (*sur lug*). Desi Sangye Gyatso (1653 – 1705), the regent of the Fifth Dalai Lama, eventually united these two schools.

Although a figure of significant scholarly and political debate even to this day, the lifework of Sangye Gyatso contributed greatly to the development of *sowa rigpa*. Not only did he oversee the creation of Tibet's first large medical university, Chagpori in Lhasa, but he also wrote and edited several medical treatises that have had a profound impact on the course of Tibetan medical knowledge and education. In the centuries predating Sangye Gyatso, scholar-physicians and medico-religious figures had added more commentaries on the *Gyushi*, writing textbooks on plant identification and the preparation of medicines. Perhaps the most significant works since the compilation of the *Gyushi* but before the time of Sangye Gyatso, was the *Oral Instruction of the Ancestor* by Zurkha Lodo Gyalpo (1509 – 1579 AD). For his part, Sangye Gyatso wrote two pivotal commentaries on the *Gyushi*, the *Blue Lapis Lazuli* and the *Amplifications,* completed in 1688 and 1691, respectively. In addition, Sangye Gyatso also commissioned the creation of a set of *thangka* scroll paintings to illustrate the *Blue Lapis Lazuli.* These paintings were not only a revolution in terms of the study of *sowa rigpa*, but also provide a fascinating perspective on the development of medical science and physiology in general. They have been reproduced in several recent publications. (See bibliography.)

The next major moment of change and revitalisation of Tibetan medicine came in the early years of the 20th century, at a time when the leadership of Tibet – the Thirteenth Dalai Lama in particular – was beginning to consider ways to modernise Tibetan society. In 1916, the Mentsikhang or 'House of Medicine and Astrology' was founded at the behest of the 13th Dalai Lama, under the direction of Khenrab Norbu (1883-1962). Unlike Chagpori, which primarily educated monk-physicians, the Mentsikhang was open to laity as well as monastics, functioning not only as a medical college and hospital, but also as a more general institute of higher education for (primarily) Tibetan nobility. The founding of the Mentsikhang itself was one of the most impressive examples of attempts by the Tibetan state to reform and modernise Tibetan society *before* the 1950s, and on their own terms. The Mentsikhang was also influenced by early 20th century Tibetan encounters with British India, including their public health measures.[6] Khenrab Norbu, who himself hailed from a renowned family of Tibetan medical practitioners, also instituted some changes to the classical Tibetan medical curriculum in an attempt to adapt *sowa rigpa* to the health care needs of Tibetans in his day.

Chagpori was destroyed during the Lhasa Uprising of 1959 against the Chinese domination in Tibet; a radio tower now stands in its place, atop the 'Iron Hill' for which this institute was named. The Mentsikhang still exists in Lhasa today. Despite the huge shifts in government policy and socio-political circumstances between pre- and post-1959 Tibet, this institution continues to operate with state support.

Tibetan Medicine and the
Rise of the People's Republic of China[7]

In order to understand how and why Tibetan medicine is taught, practiced and capitalised on in the PRC today, and before delving into deeper discussions of Tibetan medical education, production and clinical practice, we must pay some attention to the most difficult years of upheaval in Tibet's modern history and the place of *sowa rigpa* throughout this period. How did Tibetan medicine fare during the Chinese 'peaceful

---

6 The British missions to Tibet during the first 40 years of the 20th century, beginning with the 1904 Younghusband Expedition, also included the introduction of biomedicine to Tibet, first through the establishment of a medical clinic in Gyantse in 1904. See McKay (2003) for more on this topic.

7 The work of several scholars, particularly Adams, Janes, and Samuel, have been particularly helpful in framing this discussion of Tibetan medicine's more recent history (full citations in bibliography).

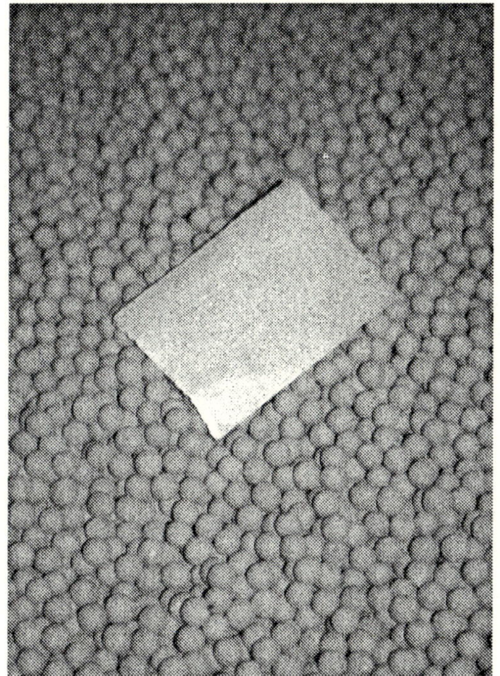

Traditionally manufactured pills   ©TIN

Medicine sale at the Potala   ©TIN

liberation' of Tibet and the subsequent years of the Cultural Revolution and changing policies, from collectivisation to privatisation, and through the development of minority nationality policies? During this ideological fraught time, what became of the deep intermingling of medical and spiritual practice? How was Tibetan medicine able to make a place for itself within the PRC's vision of national heritage and the value of minority nationalities' traditions?

Compared with many of Tibet's religious and cultural institutions, and with the blatant exception of Chagpori's destruction, Tibetan medicine is generally thought to have emerged from the ravages of the 1950s, '60s, and '70s more intact. The 'science' inherent in *sowa rigpa* has been both a blessing and a curse over the last four decades, as have the historical and mytho-historical

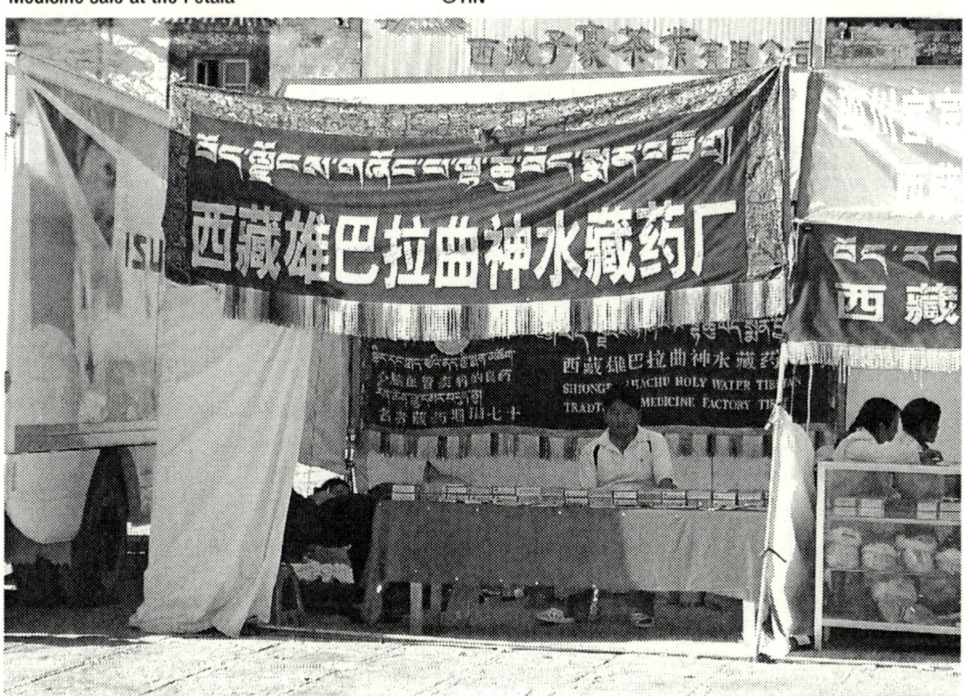

connections between traditional Chinese medicine and Tibetan medicine. These medical systems share aspects of their *pharmacopoeia*, as well as treatment techniques such as moxibustion, acupuncture, and massage. This in turn has been folded into the nationalist narratives of not only an independent Tibet and a pre-Mao China, but also into the vision of the People's Republic. As such, Tibetan medicine education and practice was 'rehabilitated' much more quickly than Buddhist ritual or many folk practices designated as 'superstitious' and 'feudal' by the PRC leadership and ideology. However, this is a relative statement. Like all of Tibet's social, religious, and political institutions, *sowa rigpa* knowledge and practice did come under attack, and was transformed in many ways during the periods from 1959 –1966, during the Cultural Revolution (1966-1976), and during the reform movements from 1978 to the present.

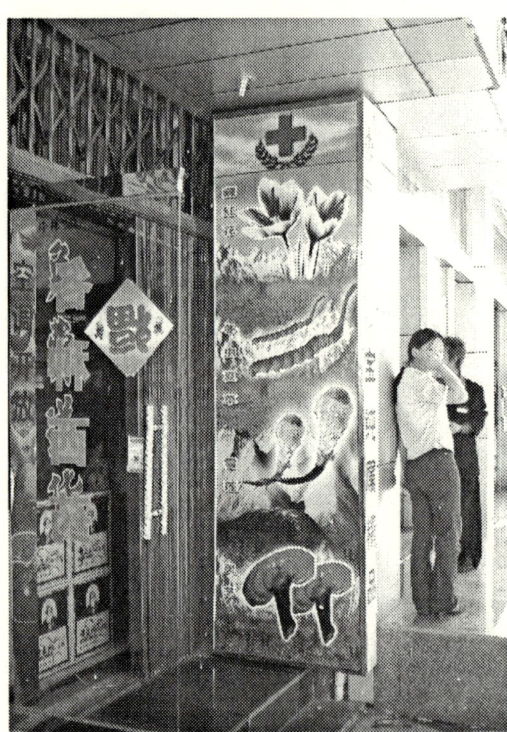

Advertisement of Tibetan medicine in Lhasa ©TIN

It is impossible to separate the changes that have befallen Tibetan medicine in contemporary China from the rise of the Chinese socialist state and the subsequent health care policies it has implemented, as well as the ways the People's Republic has both classified and controlled its 'minority nationalities' (Chinese: *minzu*) and valorised ethnomedicine, particularly as Traditional Chinese Medicine (Chinese: *zhongyi*). Furthermore, ethnomedical practices within China, including Tibetan medicine, have also existed in dialogue and sometimes conflict with biomedicine since well before the founding of the PRC.[8] During the Cultural Revolution, the Mao-led state implemented China's infamous 'barefoot doctor' model throughout the country, including the newly 'liberated' Tibet. The goal of this programme, providing basic universal health care for all citizens, was considered a lofty one both within and outside of China at the time, despite the havoc that these young and/or unskilled health care providers sometimes wreaked throughout rural communities. Yet it is important to note that this programme and other early Chinese health care policies also explicitly addressed its minority nationalities – including Tibet – by offering training in basic biomedicine and attempting to use and build on traditional medical resources.

---

8 For example, during the 1920s-30s, practitioners of *zhongyi* came under attack by biomedically trained Chinese physicians who tried to outlaw *zhongyi* practice while at the same time capitalise on traditional Chinese remedies, particularly herbal medicines. This resulted in widespread protests by *zhongyi* practitioners and the eventual establishment of state support for Traditional Chinese Medicine. See Xu (1997).

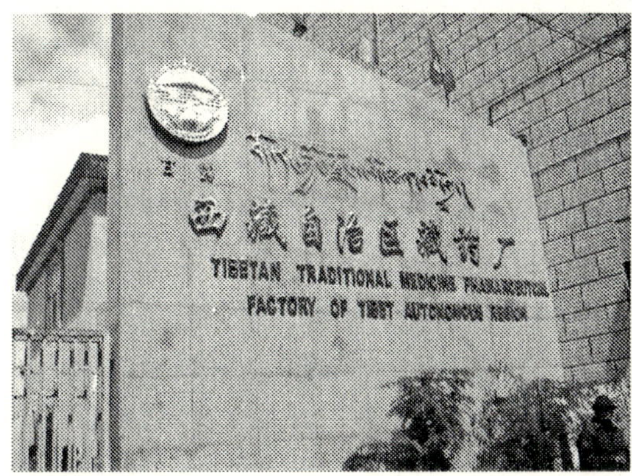
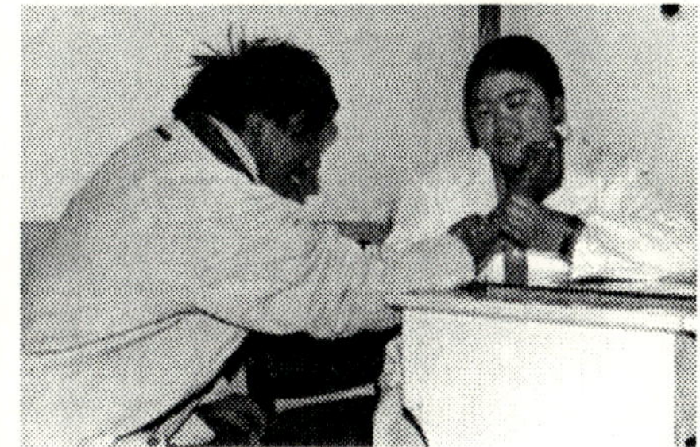

Above: Rokpa clinic in Kham   ©TIN

Left: Tibet medicine factory of TAR   ©TIN

This approach toward health care policy was also an attempt by the newly formed People's Republic to officially sanction cultural diversity through its support of medical pluralism.[9] However, it is important to note that this official tolerance of medical pluralism and, by implication, cultural diversity, was also coupled with an equally strong need to control the population, particularly minority regions. And, as in other moments in history, medicine provided a key way to do just this. Health care was provided, as it were, to loyal citizens – people whose bodies literally and figuratively stitched together the image of a coherent new People's Republic. As one scholar of Tibet has written:

> *Health care services were received from a benevolent state so long as both health care practitioners and patients continued to show unquestioned loyalty to the state's political ideology, even when that required retraining practitioners and rewriting medical theory and history.* (Adams 1999: 4)

It is in this regard that the story of Tibetan medicine most blatantly diverges from the notion of a model minority: Tibet's historical position vis-à-vis China, as well as the relationship between Buddhism and *sowa rigpa* made Tibetan medicine a more 'risky' practice than other ethnomedical practices among China's officially recognised 56 nationalities. Fundamentally, the connections between Tibetan medicine and Tibetan Buddhism posed a problem for the Chinese state. Tibetan medicine was more than a 'folk' medical tradition. It was grounded in a textual corpus with a very sophisticated medical epistemology, which in turn was intertwined with Buddhist philosophy. As such, this system of medicine, embodying a cultural logic as well as medical principles, could serve to threaten, or undermine, the power of Chinese communist ideology. Reforms during the Cultural Revolution attempted to distil those ethnomedical practices the state viewed as practical and 'scientific' on the one hand, and to purge those practices deemed 'religious' or 'superstitious' on the other. What this meant for Tibetan medicine was often the retraining of Tibet's physicians to serve the masses, imprisonment for some highly adept *sowa rigpa* practitioners or the driving underground or into exile of others.

---

9 See Farquhar (1994) and Adams (1999) for more information on this aspect of Chinese medical history.

Fundamentally, this period was marked by the Chinese government drawing an increasingly stark line between those aspects of Tibetan medical practice that were viewed as legitimate or illegitimate. Although Tibetan medicine continued to be taught and practiced during this period, it was under extremely compromised circumstances: private practice and instruction was squelched or only practiced secretly, while officially sanctioned education was stripped of anything connected to Tibetan religious practice or, in some ways more significantly, to Tibetan medical theory. Instead, *sowa rigpa* was stripped of much of its necessary complexity, often reduced to a list of disorders and treatments along a 'barefoot doctor', biomedical line. Practically speaking, this has meant that a generation of *amchi* educated at state sanctioned institutions during this time were denied a full *sowa rigpa* education – a fact that has continued to bear on current generations of students, as we shall see in Chapter Two. In addition, during the Cultural Revolution, Mentsikhang doctors as well as private practice *amchi* came under attack and lay Tibetans who were caught seeking out medico-religious treatments were subject to punishment, including physical and mental abuse. It is also important to note that the abuses faced by Tibetans, including *amchi* and their patients, did not begin or end with the Cultural Revolution. The 1959 Lhasa Uprising took place seven years before the start of the Cultural Revolution and can be seen as a reaction to the previous decade of Chinese encroachment into Tibetan social, political, economic and cultural landscapes. Likewise, the periods of reform and 'opening up' that marked the end of the Cultural Revolution for much of the rest of the PRC did not stop abuse and destruction in Tibet.

And yet, this is only half of the story. The fact that Tibetan medicine was already a state-supported enterprise under the pre-1950s Tibetan government, and that formal and informal exchanges between Tibetan *amchi* and *zhongyi* practitioners had been occurring for decades, if not for centuries, paved the way for official negotiations between Tibetan doctors, medical institutions and the Chinese state during the 1950s and beyond. Likewise, the role that Tibetan medicine played in maintaining the overall health of Tibetan populations was recognised in early PRC rhetoric and policies, and *sowa rigpa* was recognised as a member of the 'family' of Chinese medicines.[10] Ironically perhaps, one of the effects of the 1959 Tibetan Uprising and Chinese takeover of the Tibetan government was the legitimisation of Tibetan medicine under the new regime, including some government subsidies. Even during the era of violent and chaotic government doublespeak, imprisonment and destruction that defined the period from 1959 through the Cultural Revolution, Tibetan medicine and its practitioners suffered but Tibetan medicine was never stripped of its state endorsement. Later, during the period of Deng Xiaoping-sponsored reforms after 1980, Tibetan medicine experienced a significant amount of state-supported growth. The Mentsikhang became officially incorporated into the TAR Health Bureau during this time, and the Tibetan Medical College was established, gaining state support and legitimacy, first as an offshoot of the Mentsikhang, and later as an independent institution of higher learning governed by the Education Ministry of the TAR.

10 Janes (2001:199)

Contemporary Tibetan Medical Institutions

Despite the host of social, economic and political challenges faced by *amchi* today, *sowa rigpa* continues to be practiced in rural and urban settings, in vocational and professional contexts internationally: from Ladakh to Bhutan, from Amdo to South India, from Taipei to the TAR. Within the TAR and other culturally Tibetan regions of the PRC, Tibetan medicine has been officially integrated into health care policy and services, at the village, township, county, and prefecture levels since the mid-late 1980s. For instance, each of the TAR's six prefectures includes a state-run Tibetan medical hospital. Aside from Lhasa-based institutions, hospitals and factories of Tibetan medicine in places such as Nagchu Prefecture, TAR and Xining, Qinghai Province, are large and thriving. Yet several institutes of Tibetan medicine continue to define, and to a certain extent dominate, the present and future of Tibetan medicine – at least as it is officially recognised by the PRC government. Although we are most concerned with those institutions that exist inside the TAR and other ethnically Tibetan regions of the PRC, it is important to mention – and contextualise – these institutions in the light of those that have been rebuilt in exile. For, although there is very little official dialogue between these institutions, unofficially they are quite aware of each other's activities.

The Mentsikhang in Lhasa today is an official state-supported enterprise, complete with both an in-patient facility of approximately 300 beds in north Lhasa, and an out-patient facility in the Mentsikhang's original location, just down from the Barkhor marketplace

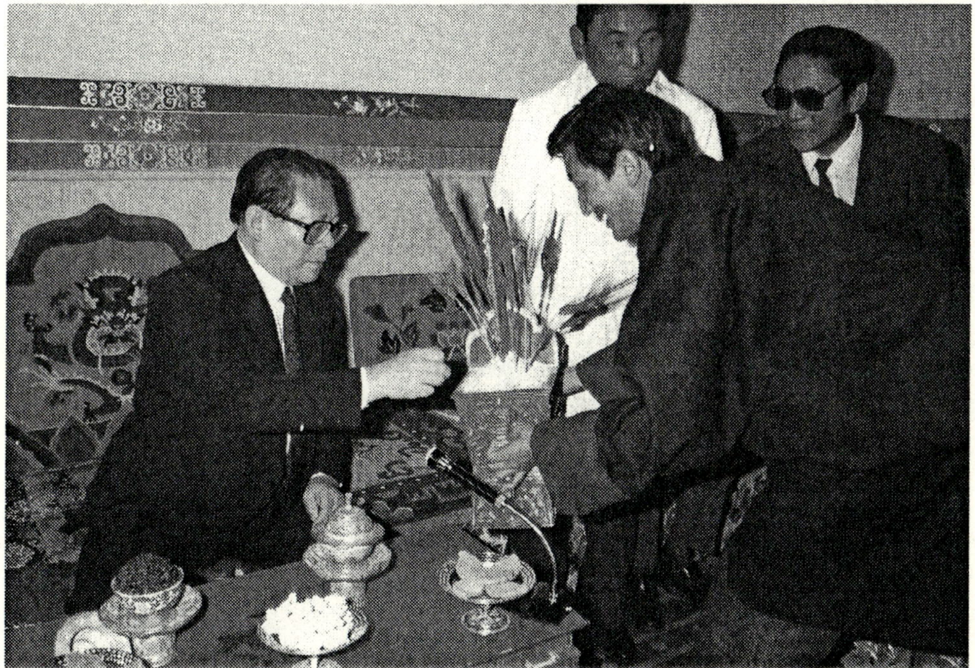

Jiang Zemin visits the Tibet Medical Hospital in Lhasa　　　　　　　　　　　　　　　　　　©TIN

and the Jokhang temple in the centre of old Lhasa. The in-patient Mentsikhang also houses a research department and, at another site, runs a for-profit medical factory. Many of the oldest and most experienced practitioners of Tibetan medicine spend a large portion of their time at the out-patient Mentsikhang. At the in-patient hospital, the work of healing has been divided up into wards that mirror those you would find in a western hospital: gastro-intestinal problems and bone problems, gynaecology, surgery, two different wards for internal medicine and one for neurological disorders, as well as specialists devoted to liver and kidney disorders. The two branches of the hospital also house both a Tibetan medical and a biomedical pharmacy. As the largest official Tibetan medical hospital in the TAR, the Mentsikhang is a major hub for the distribution of Tibetan medicines to remote areas of the TAR. It also maintains links with other county and prefecture-level Tibetan medical hospitals in other Chinese provinces with significant Tibetan populations, notably in Qinghai and Sichuan, as well as in Chamdo, at the eastern edge of the TAR, and Nagchu Prefecture, which encompasses much of the Chang Tang or 'Northern Plains' of Tibet, home to many of the TAR's nomadic communities. Significantly, clinicians and administrators at the Mentsikhang estimate that eighty to ninety percent of their patients are Tibetan, whereas at many of the other hospitals in Lhasa the patient profiles include more Chinese immigrants. The Mentsikhang also operates on a sliding scale of payment and does not turn away patients who do not have the ability to pay their medical bills – a reality that is not the case in some of Lhasa's other hospitals. The Mentsikhang administration and staff foster a strong relationship between their in-patient and out-patient facilities, which is critical for tracking illnesses and recoveries. Many of the younger physicians at both the in-patient and the out-patient hospital are graduates from the Tibetan Medical College.

This brings us to the other major institution of Tibetan medicine, and a hub for the present and future of this practice in another sense: the Tibetan Medical College. The

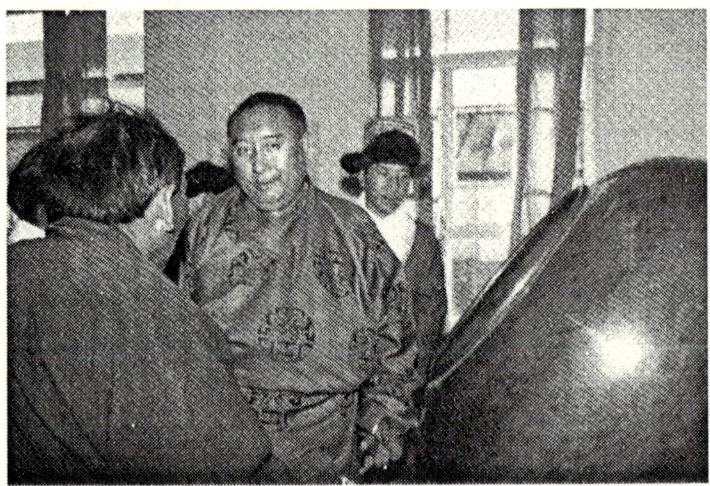

The late Panchen Lama visiting a Tibetan medicine factory   ©TIN

institution began as the Tibetan Medicine College of Tibet University – a combination of the Tibetan Medicine School, established in 1983, and the Tibetan Medicine Department, established in 1985. The Tibetan Medical College became a separate institute under the Education Bureau in 1993, and is now located in north Lhasa. The college includes nine departments, including a medicine factory and a research department. Details of the curriculum at this institution and others will be discussed in Chapter Two. Here, suffice to say that this institution is more of an academic than a clinical establishment or a teaching hospital, although students in the various degree programmes are provided with clinical as well as theoretical experience. The Tibetan Medical College is considered by many Tibetans to be the premier *sowa rigpa* teaching institution. Many graduates of the Tibetan Medical College go on to practice at either the Mentsikhang, at one of its branch establishments or as Tibetan doctors at county and township level clinics throughout the TAR and other culturally Tibetan areas of the PRC. In addition to these Lhasa-based institutions, a number of county and prefecture level hospitals and institutes of Tibetan medicine exist in the TAR and in Kham and Amdo, particularly in and around Derge, Chamdo, Xining, and Labrang, as well as the Kongpo and Nagchu regions of the TAR. The Qinghai College of Tibetan Medicine, in Xining, is a particularly thriving institution, with more than 600 students. Likewise, the Labrang monastery also includes a prosperous Tibetan medical college, clinic, and factory. The Central University for Nationalities in Beijing also includes a Tibetan Medicine Institute, within the College of Life and Environmental Sciences.

The other two institutions of Tibetan medicine that are worth describing in some detail are the Men-tsee-khang in Dharamsala, India, and the Chagpori Medical Institute in Darjeeling. Although they are located outside the PRC, these institutions on the south side of the Himalayas are not only aware of their counterparts to the north, but the relationship between them also bears on how Tibetan medicine is represented and practiced in other countries, what Tibetan medical research entails and how Tibetan

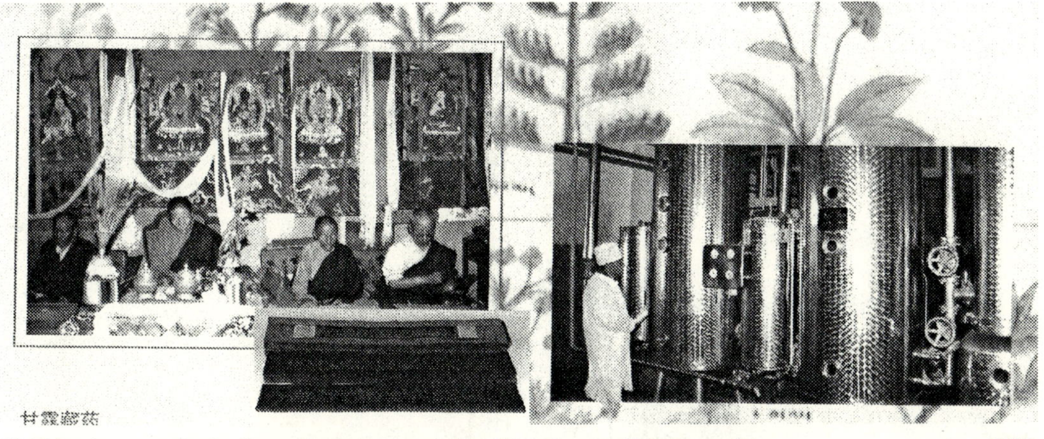

Official brochures emphasise the continuity between 'old' and 'new' ways of Tibetan medicine   ©TIN

medicines themselves are sold and consumed on the world market. The links – or sometimes the lack of official connections – between those institutes in Tibet and those in exile also bear directly on the future of Tibetan medical practice and the education of future generations of physicians, as we will discuss in more detail in Chapter Two.

The Men-tsee-khang is the official reproduction of the Lhasa Mentsikhang in exile. Established in 1961, the Men-tsee-khang is endorsed by the private office of the Dalai Lama. Unlike the developments in Lhasa, in which the Mentsikhang is primarily a clinical hospital and a for-profit medical factory, the Men-tsee-khang is both a clinical and a teaching institution. Like both the Mentsikhang and the Tibetan Medical College, the Men-tsee-khang has an active research department and a medical factory that produces medicines, which are then sold to branch clinics and private practitioners, as well as a line of beauty products called Sorig.™ Although biomedical training or clinical practice is not a part of the Men-tsee-khang's institutional philosophy, it maintains a close

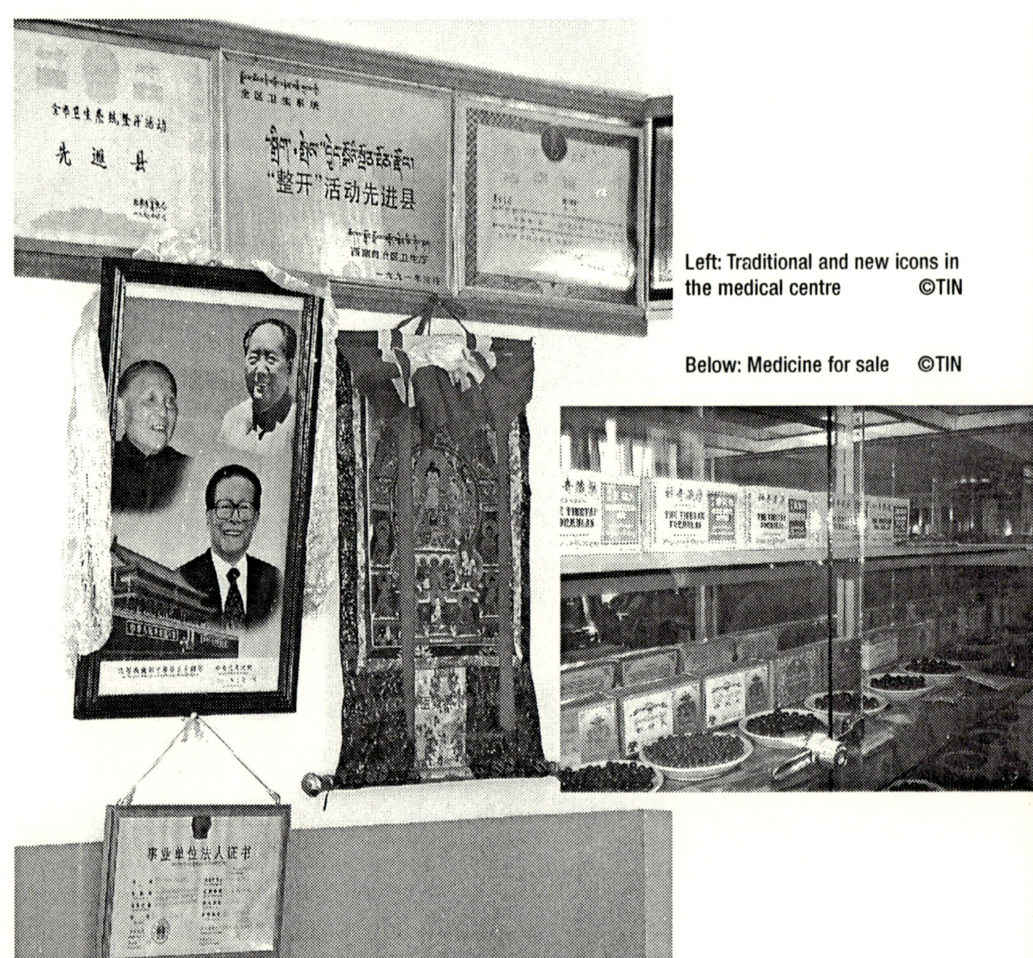

Left: Traditional and new icons in the medical centre ©TIN

Below: Medicine for sale ©TIN

relationship with the Deleg Hospital, a biomedical facility in Dharamsala. Likewise, research methodology at the Met-tsee-khang, as in parallel institutions in Tibet, is influenced by biomedicine and western scientific method. Upon graduation from the Men-tsee-khang's five-year clinical training program, students are often sent to work for branch Men-tsee-khang clinics and factories throughout India and Nepal, while some go on to teach and practice at the Men-tsee-khang itself; others go into private practice either in India or abroad. A few graduates have returned to Tibet.[11]

After the original Chagpori Institute was destroyed in 1959, this institution and the lineage of *sowa rigpa* practice it represented continued in a sporadic, informal way among private physicians and, to a certain extent, was incorporated into the founding of the Men-tsee-khang. However, in 1992, the Chagpori Medical Institute was formally re-established in exile, in the old British hill station of Darjeeling, West Bengal. The founder of this new Chagpori Medical Institute was Trogawa Rinpoche, who, aside from being an important religious figure in the world of contemporary Tibetan Buddhism, is also an *amchi* of great renown. Today, the Institute functions as both a teaching and a clinical institution, and has a small medical factory on-site. Students come from both lay and monastic backgrounds and in recent years, Trogawa Rinpoche has shown his commitment to educating Tibetan Buddhist nuns in the science and art of *sowa rigpa.* Like the Men-tsee-khang, Chagpori also occasionally hosts seminars on Tibetan medicine, astrology, language and culture for foreigners. Although Chagpori is essentially an autonomous teaching institution, the content of final examinations as well as the issuance of certificates and licenses to graduates of Chagpori are still in accordance with Men-tsee-khang standards and regulations.

Although many aspects of these exile Tibetan medical institutions are very different from those in Tibetan areas of the PRC, in other ways they continue to mirror each other. For example, the Mentsikhang in Lhasa and the Men-tsee-khang in Dharamsala are essentially state-run institutions, which both make profits by selling medicines and other products to domestic and foreign clientele. Lay practitioners of *sowa rigpa* also outnumber monastic practitioners in both places. Although today's Chagpori has no direct Tibetan counterpart, the form and structure of the education provided there follows more closely the historical Chagpori curriculum; the institute continues to place more emphasis on the relationship between *sowa rigpa* practice and spiritual practice and many more of its students are monks or other practicing religious specialists.

Finally, after this brief discussion of influential Tibetan medicine institutions, it is important to reiterate that for many centuries, Tibetan medicine was not *primarily* taught through large schools such as the original Chagpori, but rather was a body of knowledge passed down through religious or hereditary lineage, through a combination of oral and literary sources. In fact, to distinguish the early 'schools' of Tibetan medicine from the sense that master teachers were also key 'lineage holders' is to miss the ways that these modes of knowing Tibetan medicine were – and still are – fundamentally connected. Particularly in Tibetan areas of the PRC, however, it is not

---

11 The Men-tsee-khang maintains an informative website: www.men-tsee-khang.org.

necessary or possible for all *amchi* to also act as religious specialists in fulfilling their role as healers. Yet it is also important to recognise that religious and medical practice need not be intertwined; indeed many contemporary practitioners of *sowa rigpa* both in Tibet and in exile stress a separation of religious from medical expertise. In other words, *sowa rigpa* can be construed by state policy or by *amchi* themselves as a technical practice in which the religious dimension is not fundamental to successful healing. Yet many *amchi* would say these links to medico-religious lineage remain crucial to the social legitimacy of a Tibetan medical practitioner to this day, even though this connection is being challenged by a variety of social, economic and political changes, as we shall explore in later chapters.

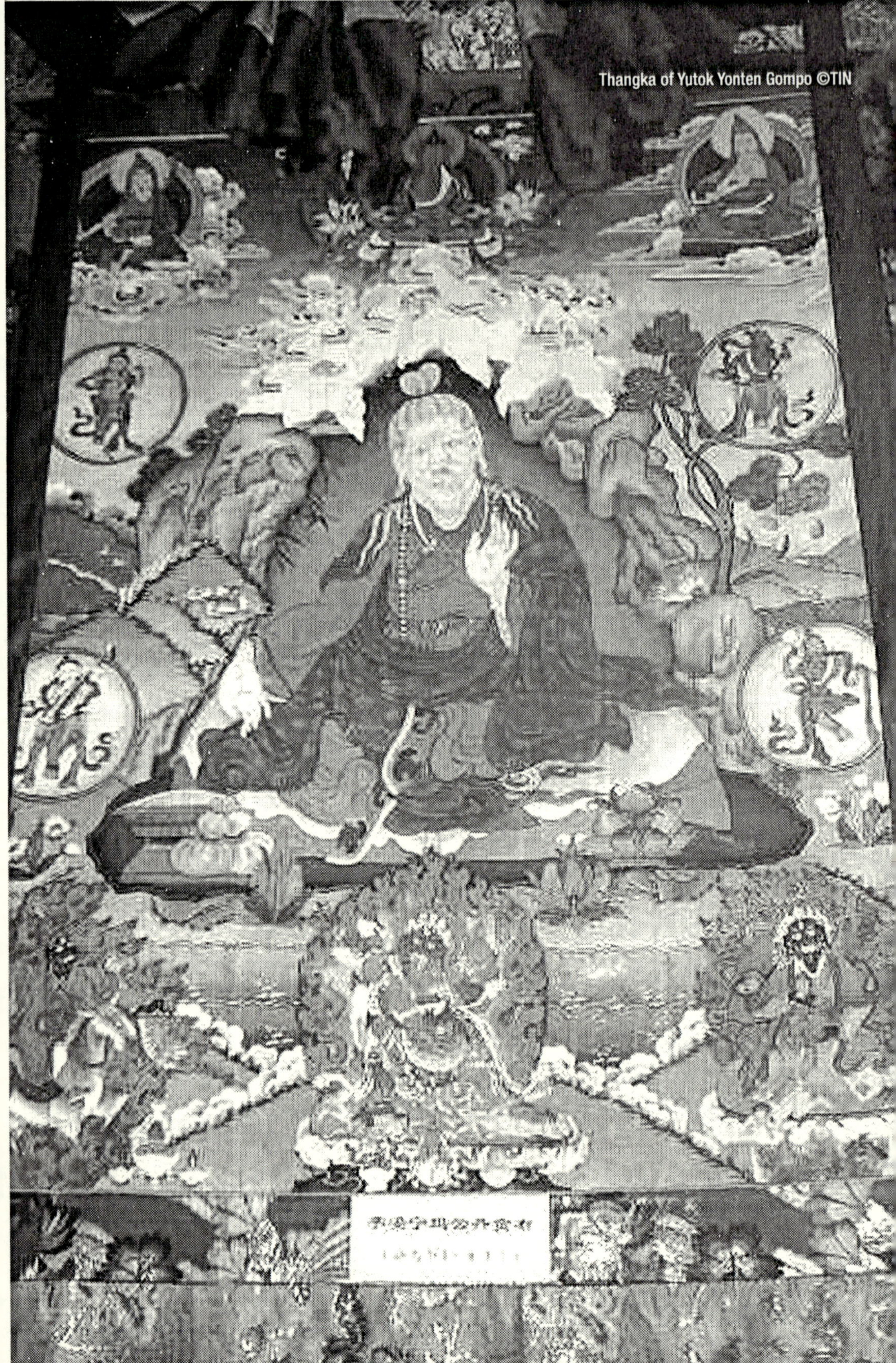
Thangka of Yutok Yonten Gompo ©TIN

Chapter Two

The Transmission of Knowledge: Tibetan Medical Education

As we have seen in Chapter One, many different models of Tibetan medical education and practice have existed throughout the course of *sowa rigpa* history: from master-apprentice relationships that last for decades or generations, to institutional programmes with set syllabi and certification procedures, and everything in between. It is important to de-emphasise an idealised classical model of Tibetan medical education, or to create too stark a divide between private, lineage-based instruction and institutional learning. While such distinctions are important, and reflect larger social, economic, and political changes inside Tibet, we should not see them as mutually exclusive, either historically or in the present. Instead, we hope to show something of the diversity of practices that we find in Tibetan regions of the PRC today.

Medical education is integrally tied to the clinical practice of Tibetan medicine. It is also linked directly to the survival of Tibet's rich cultural, scientific, linguistic, and religious heritage. Simply put, how a society is able to educate its people and, in that sense, pass down cultural knowledge, bears directly on the future of that society. Education, medical or otherwise, is the vehicle by which cultures can change and also sustain themselves. In this sense, a study of Tibetan medicine can reveal some of the ways that Tibetan identity within the PRC is constructed and experienced. The issue of curriculum within Tibetan medical education – what and how to teach, whether or not to introduce biomedicine into Tibetan medical courses, what the relationship is and should be between institutional and lineage-based master-apprentice pedagogy – plays out at the level of large, state-supported, (or state-in-exile supported,) institutes for Tibetan medicine in the PRC and India. But these issues are also having crucial impacts on the future of smaller, private schools of *sowa rigpa*, both within the PRC and in regions such as Ladakh, India, northern Nepal or even Bhutan and Mongolia. They also bear on the realm of private, informal instruction if only because they have an impact on how both patients and novice *amchi* conceive of medical expertise. In this sense, the changes occurring within Tibetan medical education are not unique to those institutions in the PRC but are part of larger movements and pressures to standardise and 'modernise' Tibetan medicine, to garner state and international support, to tap into the transnational interest in 'alternative' therapies, and to allow *amchi* to survive in market economies. Yet the strictures of Tibetan medical education inside the PRC diverge in specific ways from *sowa rigpa* schools in exile or in other national contexts. Fundamentally, the forms and content of *sowa rigpa* education bear directly on the health and well being of Tibetans now and in the future. Indeed, how one comes to know the mind and body, and know how to alleviate suffering, cuts to the core of personal and collective identity.

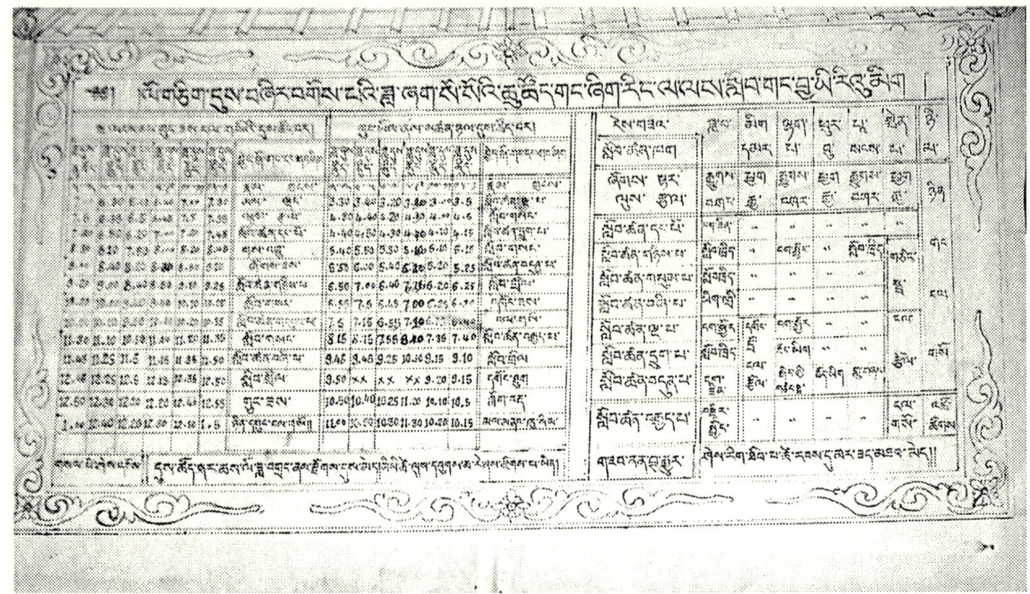

Curriculum ©TIN

In relation to the large, state supported institutions of Tibetan medicine – specifically the Mentsikhang and the Tibetan Medical College – the path of becoming a Tibetan doctor is not much different from that of earning other sorts of university and advanced degrees, at least in how a student's time and, to a large extent, motivation, is configured. It is one of many educational and, eventually, professional paths. However, Tibetan medical education does differ from other avenues for higher education in one fundamental respect: it is the only university and post-graduate course of study in which the primary language of pedagogy remains Tibetan, as opposed to Chinese. As in historical Tibet, today's *sowa rigpa* education retains an emphasis on Tibetan literary competence, memorisation of medical texts, identification of plants, etc. Yet there is an increasing emphasis on biomedicine and a need for Chinese linguistic competence in many Tibetan medicine institutes, both state-sponsored and private. This is justified in terms of the need to adhere to professional standards and clinical competency, and to distinguish between kinds of practitioners, through certification and licensing. But it is also part of a future vision of Tibetan medicine in which the medicines themselves, as well as processes of diagnosis and treatment, are seen as scientifically on par with biomedicine as it is practiced in China and internationally.

Even though aspects of the 'traditional' *sowa rigpa* curriculum have been rewritten over the centuries, as well as the last four decades, both Tibetan practitioners/teachers and the Chinese state rely on the title 'Traditional Tibetan Medicine' to describe this system of healing. At one level, this is simple and strategic. Parallels can then be drawn and state support justified between Tibetan medicine and Traditional Chinese Medicine (TCM, Chinese: *zhongyi*). During the late 1970s-early 1980s reform movements in the PRC, the rewriting of curricula have also meant the re-inclusion of parts of the *Gyushi* as well as other medico-religious texts that were banned during the Cultural Revolution. In that sense, there has been a return, or a revitalisation, of certain 'traditional' aspects of Tibetan medical education and practice over the past two decades. But this 'revitalisation' is partial and fragmented, and depends to a large extent on the presence of adept teachers who can guide students through these texts.

In a more general sense, though, this need to defend and yet transform what is meant by 'tradition' – particularly in the context of Tibetan medical education – is not unique to *sowa rigpa* practice in the TAR. Similar discussions about what 'traditional Tibetan medicine' means are currently being debated among practitioners of *sowa rigpa* in Ladakh, Nepal, Mongolia, Bhutan and of course at institutions such as the Dharamsala Men-tsee-khang. The use of the term 'traditional' in relation to Tibetan medicine also surfaces in the context of practitioners of *sowa rigpa* lobbying for state and NGO support in a variety of national contexts. Indeed, we could see this need to defend and yet transform so-called traditional practices as a fundamental component of what it means to be modern. This issue also cuts to the core of what it means for a young person to be shaped by educational experiences and modes of knowing, and how this, in turn, shapes a society's future.

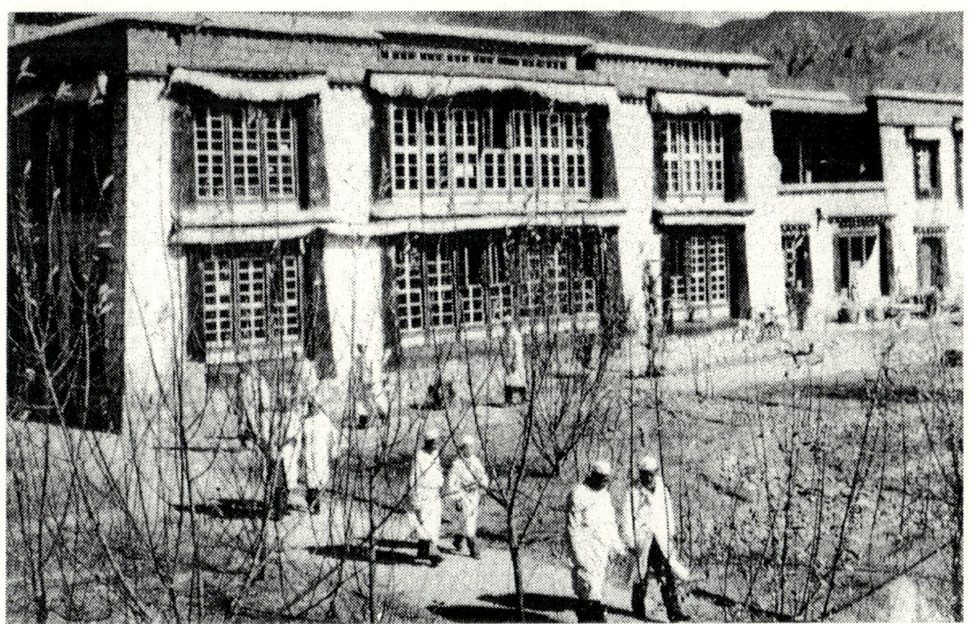

Former premises of the Tibet Medical Hospital, Lhasa   ©TIN

Education Reforms and State Institutions

A Tibetan medical doctor from Lhasa summarised the history and current circumstances of Tibetan medical institutions as follows:

> *We must start by saying that here in Tibet, our medicine, nectar of the gods, comes from the Potala and from Lhasa. Historically, there were amchi from many places in Tibet, but they did not work together. For example, there were schools of sowa rigpa established at Drigung, at the Potala and in Shigatse but they remained [separate]. After this, Desi Sangye Gyatso founded Chagpori. The main motivation for establishing this school was to combine and improve all the different aspects of Tibetan Medicine, and to make a place for a mentsikhang, a school, and a place to do research. They also chose Chagpori because the iron hill was the best suited, environmentally, to making medicines that were most powerful.*
>
> *After Chagpori was made no more, many people came from that institution to the Mentsikhang. At that time, the Norbulingkha also had lha men pa [literally 'deity physicians'] as did Samye and Tsurphu, Drepung, and other monasteries and places of study. They all came to the Mentsikhang after that time. After some hardship, the Mentsikhang began to flourish. We treated patients, did research, and also provided clinical practice to amchi who were studying. Eventually, we realised that we also had to start a factory, for the development of Tibetan medicine. So, we started a small factory in the 1970s, and then by the 1980s it was getting bigger. Now there are many factories aside from ours (...) But since Chagpori was no longer, we needed a good medical school. For some time, there was a school of Tibetan medicine at the Barkhor, which was connected to the Mentsikhang. This is where I learned. But that was not adequate for the future of Tibetan medicine, and so we needed to make a place that was specifically for study. We decided to make the Mentsikhang and the Tibetan Medical College separate, and this was how things went in 1988-89, until the present. Now the Tibetan Medical College comes under the Education Bureau, while the Mentsikhang is governed by the Health Bureau.*

It seems fitting to begin this discussion of educational reforms and today's schools of *sowa rigpa* with this reflection – a reconstruction of history that casts the trajectory of Tibetan medicine as an unbroken lineage of teaching and healing on the one hand, and also as a system that, both before the Chinese annexation of Tibet and after, has experienced radical shifts. As this doctor is speaking from Lhasa, events such as the destruction of Chagpori are glossed over and repressed in favour of a depiction of continuity, as well as specialisation and development within Tibetan medical education and practice. Likewise, the separation of the Mentsikhang from the Tibetan Medical College in Lhasa is portrayed as depoliticised and inevitable, whereas the history of this division is much more complicated; these contemporary institutions are quite

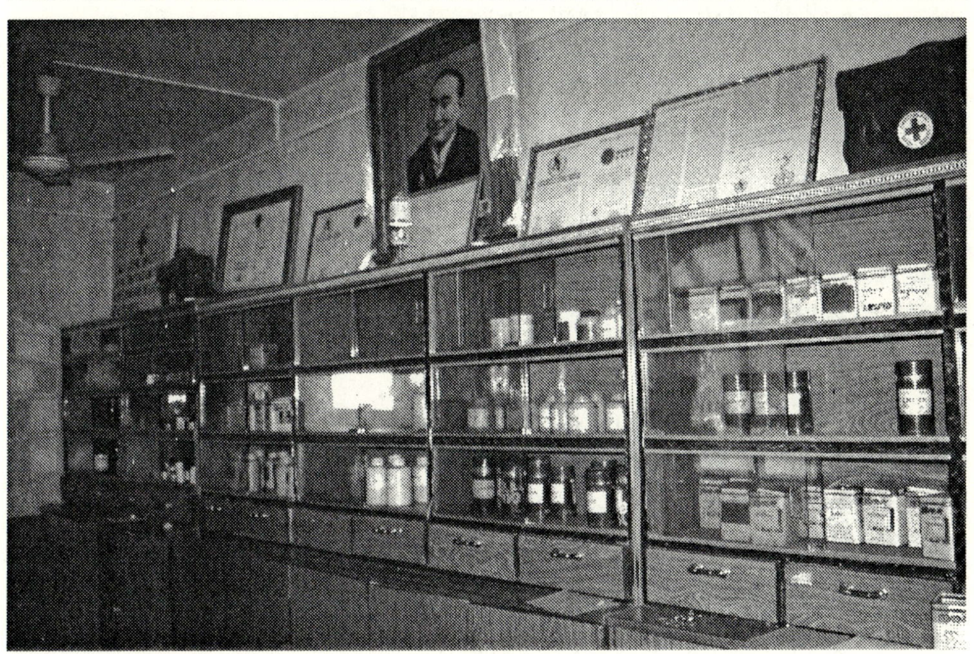

Monastery dispensary   ©TIN

competitive with each other, despite the ways they also rely on each other. The other thing to notice about this *amchi*'s historical reflections is how he connects particular places to different schools of medicine, as well as an environmental awareness that links the teaching of *sowa rigpa* and the production of medicines to well-suited places. These two themes – the importance of ecology and the value of lineage – continue to play a crucial role in what it means to become a Tibetan doctor today. They are also aspects of *sowa rigpa* education and practice that are under threat.

Although in historical times a student of Tibetan medicine might have studied for more than a decade with a master, courses of study today, both in Tibet and in exile, generally run for five to six years, with an end exam that includes both oral and written components. Memorisation of parts of the *Gyushi*, study of commentaries written from the 11th – 21st century, and oral instruction from primary and secondary teachers also continues, under varied circumstances. Programmes in Tibetan medicine expose students to clinical diagnosis experience as well as experience in plant identification and preparation of medicines; most programmes include summer trips to rural areas to identify and gather ingredients. Historically, students were expected to also have pharmacological expertise – many master Tibetan physicians devoted up to three years of their training just to pharmacology. However, this aspect of medical education, as well as the emphasis on spiritual training, no longer garner the same institutional attention, either in Tibet or in exile, although for different reasons and as a result of distinct social and political pressures, though both inherently connected to ideas about what constitutes a 'modern' life.

One of the most striking elements of change to occur since the late 1970s has been the rehabilitation of certain medical (and medico-religious) texts into the curricula taught at state institutions, and the later reprinting of the *Gyushi* and other medical texts by prominent state-run publishing houses in the TAR and other provinces of China. Along with professors and practitioners of Tibetan medicine from the Qinghai Academy of Tibetan Medicine, the Tibetan Medicine Institute at the Central University for Nationalities in Beijing and several private-practice or retired Tibetan physicians, select *amchi* associated with the Tibetan Medical College have recently participated in the creation of a new series of Tibetan medical textbooks, as well as a series of biomedical textbooks translated from Chinese into Tibetan for use within institutes of Tibetan medicine throughout the PRC.

In and around Lhasa, one will sometimes encounter an air of fear, secrecy, or simple disavowal when asking training students in aspects of *sowa rigpa* that might be categorised as 'religious' as opposed to 'scientific.' Students at the Tibetan Medical College, for instance, are not officially instructed in the *mantra*, or religious chants, used to empower medicines, although some students seek out such oral instruction privately. That being said, the quality of medical education one can receive at the state-supported institutes of Tibetan medicine is quite high, and is one of the few venues in the contemporary educational structure that allows one to focus on Tibetan language,

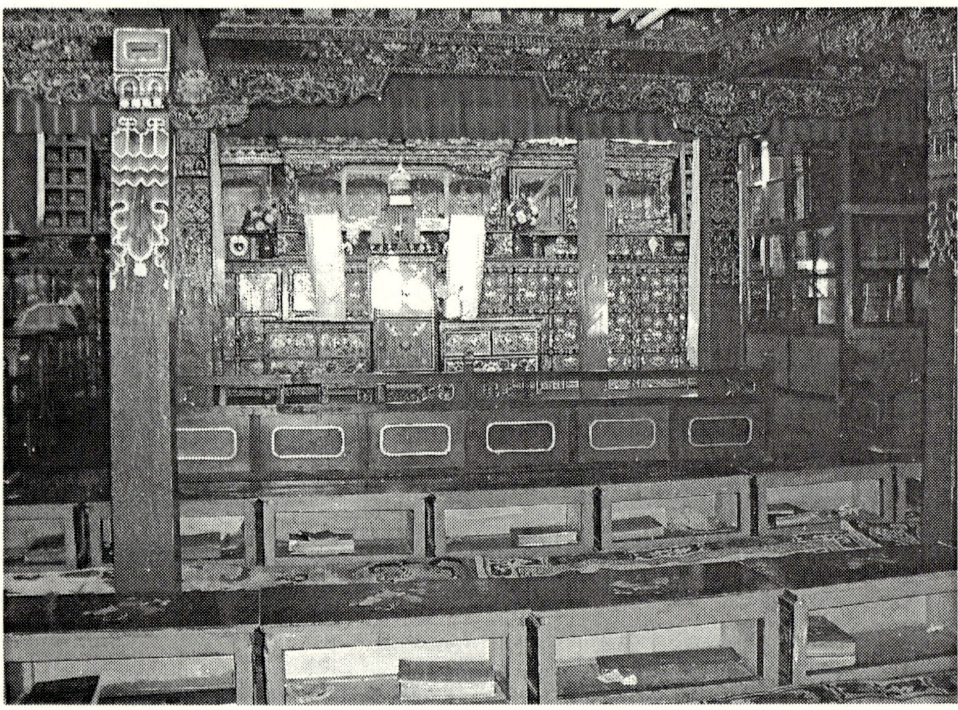

Altar at Medicine school   ©TIN

literature and grammar as a valid and valued scholastic pursuit. In addition, there is still variation within this aspect of Tibetan medical education, particularly between institutional or formalised programmes and those systems of *sowa rigpa* education that are private and informal, both in rural and urban settings.

An *amchi* who graduated from the Qinghai Academy of Tibetan Medicine, who has since moved to Lhasa and now teaches at the Tibetan Medical College, summarised some of the changes occurring within Tibetan medical education as follows:

> *In most colleges, students don't get all that much clinical experience – at least not enough to be considered a really skilled doctor. Some get this soon after, in a variety of clinical settings, but many more get channelled into other tracks, like marketing or producing medicines. But those who produce medicines also might not have more than a basic sense of the plants and other ingredients themselves, or at least not much practical experience collecting. They become more like pharmacists and marketing specialists, rather than healers. The same is true for teaching. You go through training only to arrive at the other side to be weighed down with teaching responsibilities and not a lot of time to test your own practice, your own knowledge.*

The specialisation about which this *amchi* speaks is not necessarily legislated or certified, in that students are graduating with similar, if not the same, degrees. Rather, it is part of the larger process of desegregation and specialisation that distinguishes those producing Tibetan medicine from those teaching and those prescribing Tibetan medicine as distinct entities, at least officially.

The education one receives at the Tibetan Medical College in Lhasa is considered to be one of the best within the PRC. The College includes a clinic and a medical factory, and has a population of approximately 200 students at any given time. The College offers several different types of degrees and courses. The standard curriculum to earn a bachelor's degree (*Durapa*) in Tibetan medicine lasts five years. In addition to study of the *Gyushi* and other classical medical texts, this curriculum requires that students are literate in Chinese and also exposes them to principles of biomedical anatomy and physiology, and to clinical rotations at the Mentsikhang and at Lhasa's biomedical hospitals, as well as at the Mentsikhang Factory. The College also offers a three-year course, which is favoured by students coming to the college from more rural areas, particularly those who have already had some previous medical training, (either in Tibetan medicine or biomedicine). Students in both programmes are still expected to memorise passages from the *Gyushi*, and examinations combine oral and written tests of their knowledge; however, the amount of text that students must commit to memory has decreased over time, marking a shift in not only how students learn, but also how they retain and draw on theoretical knowledge during the course of clinical practice.
In addition to these standard courses, students can also earn a Master's degree (*Kachopa*) in Tibetan medicine. In 1998, the College gained approval from the Academic

Degree Office of the State Council to offer this higher education degree – the first such institute to offer an advanced degree in Tibetan medicine. This is a three-year degree programme that includes one and a half years of didactic classroom study, followed by one and a half years during which students conduct research and write a thesis. Those students who choose to focus their research on more theoretical topics – such as an explication of the three humours, a study in pulse diagnosis, or an examination of the cause of a particular illness – usually seek out supervisors among the professors at the College. Those who choose to focus their research in a clinical setting often turn toward the Mentsikhang, both for supervision and for patient populations on which to carry out their research.

Many students complain that they do not have access to enough master physicians and teachers from whom to seek guidance – a function both of the number of elder generation *amchi* who have either passed away or passed into exile, as well as the results of the years during the Cultural Revolution when Tibetan medical education was severely compromised due to the rewriting of its texts and the banishment of anything overtly 'religious' or 'theoretical' from the curriculum. In addition, much of the research that is produced tends to be only superficially creative or analytic: the mirroring of a western academic form, or a Tibetan Buddhist mimesis, without much deep exploration within either a western scientific framework or Tibetan medical epistemology. These circumstances will, no doubt, continue to change over the coming generation –through the growing numbers and kinds of collaboration between western and Tibetan scientists and medical practitioners, and through discussions within communities of *sowa rigpa* practitioners throughout the PRC and abroad.

Experimentation, particularly in the production of new medicines, has been integral to *sowa rigpa* through the centuries. However, this focus on the production of individual research marks a distinct departure from classical Tibetan medical education. Likewise, though many of the College's students are interested in research as a means to expand their ability to treat a variety of ailments with Tibetan medicine, the connection between healer and patient becomes secondary in many instances. The standard five-year curriculum adheres most closely to a classical curriculum, in which the focus is on memorisation of medical texts, plant identification and collection, and diagnostic techniques. However, the structure of this college-level education can promote, by accident or design, a passive learning environment in which the 'right motivation' or altruism that defines a Buddhist rationale for becoming an *amchi* is secondary to the more mundane concerns of passing exams and finding a job after graduation. This is not always the case but it constitutes a trend voiced by many who have gone through the College or equivalent institutions. Although the numbers of students is small compared with most general colleges or universities within and outside the TAR, the Tibetan Medical College graduates many novice physicians, in a highly professionalised context, not all of whom will be able to find employment as Tibetan doctors in the future. Some will become the future managers of medical factories, others might be sent to work at township clinics or county hospitals, while others still will turn to teaching. But the relationship between this elite urban institution and the rural communities it serves will continue to change over time. One of the most striking elements of this state-supported education structure is the way that it is creating a generation of Tibetan physicians who are theoretically adept and sometimes quite specialised in their knowledge, but who do not necessarily have a practical knowledge of Tibetan medical plants, and who sometimes graduate with very little clinical experience, before being sent out to practice.

The Mentsikhang is no longer primarily a teaching institution, but it does provide medical training on a more vocational model to students with basic formal education, as well as to a small number of monks and nuns who, after completion of their one to two year apprenticeship, are expected to return to their monastic institutions and serve as health care providers. This model of education cum clinical practice also exists at Mentsikhang branch hospitals in other parts of the TAR, as well as in county-level Tibetan medical hospitals throughout Kham and Amdo. In Lhasa, these Mentsikhang apprenticeships are focused at the out-patient institution, and appeal to students who have fewer financial resources and, in some cases, less knowledge of spoken and written Chinese than those at the Tibetan Medical College. The model of education in this instance is a hybrid between a classical master-apprentice relationship, in which the principal form of knowledge transmission is oral instruction, supplemented by textual study and hands-on experience, and a Tibetan version of biomedical paramedic or Emergency Medical Technician (EMT) training. The benefits of this model of training are twofold. First, young students gain access to some of the foremost Tibetan doctors still alive and practicing today. Second, they begin their education with a strong connection to patients and clinical experience – something that many graduates from the Tibetan Medical College experience less of before graduation. Students who follow this path might go on to study at the Tibetan Medical College or other comparable institutions in their home regions outside the TAR.

The other large, state-run institution of Tibetan medical education worth mentioning is the Qinghai Medical Academy and Hospital in Xining. The Qinghai Medical Academy was founded in 1988. The college includes six departments – administration, education/curriculum, Tibetan medicine, Tibetan drugs, research and clinical care – and the opportunity for students to major either in Tibetan medical practice or Tibetan medical pharmacology and medicinal drugs. At present there are more than 600 students who have gone through this college's course, or who are currently enrolled. The Academy also includes an in-house medical factory for use in the hospital.

Private Instruction, Lineage, and Medico-Religious Practice

The far wall of the Tibetan Medical College library is dominated by a large *thangka* painting that depicts the history and key lineages in Tibetan medical practice. It is a depiction of myth, religion and history, one that moves through space as well as time, and that marks in ink and earthen pigment, gold leaf and semi-precious stone, what many consider the jewels of *sowa rigpa* teaching and practice. Sangye Menla, the Medicine Buddha, sits in meditative repose at the top of the canvas, surrounded by protector deities and *bodhisattva*. Further down the painting, characters such as Yuthog Yonten Gompo the Elder and the founders of the Northern and Southern schools rest. Below this is a depiction of Chagpori and the Mentsikhang. The fact that this painting hangs in this premier institution of Tibetan medical learning also hints at the somewhat false divide between private, lineage-based instruction and large-scale institutional learning in Tibetan medical history and current practice. Tibetan medicine has evolved through a series of master healers passing on their knowledge to student disciples, but also through the schools they established, the institutions they formed and the modes of knowledge transmission they practiced. And yet, this relationship between lineage and institution, between private and public instruction, is one of the elements of Tibetan medical education that has changed most since 1959. This is due in part to the ramifications of Chinese state modernisation policies, and explicit campaigns against 'superstition' and 'backwards' tradition, including medico-religious teachings, and in part a result of more overarching yet subtle shifts in population, urban/rural dynamics, and access to learned teachers. As mentioned above, many of Tibet's most skilled physicians suffered during the Cultural Revolution and many have made their way into exile over the past four decades. Others continue to practice in Tibet, under a variety of circumstances, some as private physicians, some as state employees or some who retire from a lifetime of civil service only to open private clinics and take on students.

Such diversity is acknowledged, but one of the net results of this trend toward institutionalised learning is a decline in the perpetuation of a more holistic model of *sowa rigpa*. This includes forms of knowledge transmitted solely through medico-spiritual initiations, empowerments and other orally transmitted tantric medical practices, (*loong, wang and men ngag,*) as well as a model of education in which theoretical knowledge and practical skill are encouraged simultaneously. These latter modes of learning allow novice *amchi* to establish his or her reputation and build confidence not only in diagnosis and treatment but also in pharmacology and the preparation of medicines. Although such instruction and practice does continue, it is becoming increasingly rare both within the PRC and in exile. Yet *sowa rigpa* practitioners who have had such training remain highly valued by rural and urban Tibetans alike. When one begins to ask Tibetans, whether laypeople or monastics, doctors or not, about who they consider the most skilled *amchi*, stories begin to filter out about such private practitioners, tales that not only echo a Tibetan past but that also attest to the Tibetan present.

Although many people will also cite the growing fame of Tibetan medicine throughout the world as a testament to the Mentsikhang's reputation, or express awe at the fortunes made by selling particular Tibetan medicines in mainland China and abroad, Tibetans often value private physicians and medico-religious specialists precisely because theirs is a non-institutionalised practice. Lineage-based medical expertise tends toward knowledge and practices that have been passed down from father to son, uncle to nephew, or from root teacher to disciple, and whose efficacy derives as much from a practitioners' diagnostic skill and methods of producing medicines as from the weight and power of this lineage history itself. Such relationships also illustrate the connection between lineage and particular areas of medical expertise. Some private lineage *amchi* will specialise in certain kinds of medicines or therapies and will pass on not only this technical skill – such as golden needle acupuncture or bone setting – but also a sense of authority and trust vested in this line of healers by patients themselves. Some private practitioners have often explicitly disassociated their practices from the Chinese state and have sometimes suffered the consequences. Part of the efficacy of this sort of practice is political in nature: a choice against being absorbed into or restricted by the Chinese health care system, or against making medicines in a mechanised and 'standardised' way.

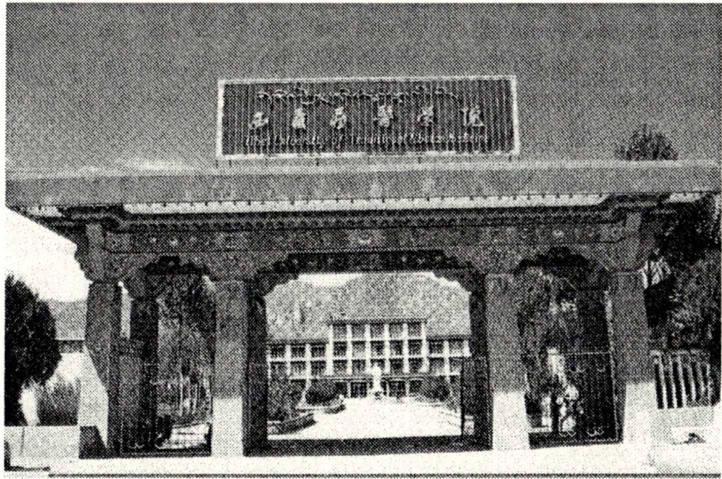

Gate of the Tibet
University of Traditional
Tibetan Medicine, Lhasa
©TIN

Yet many practitioners at both private clinics and state-run institutions will say that lineage should not be considered a criterion for whether or nor one can become a skilled *amchi*. Indeed, some Tibetans view this notion as an 'old' way of thinking; one that does not take into account the populist-cum-state communist notion that class or heritage should not determine one's profession, and that there are many ways to serve the masses. Others cite the inherent bias against women within a more traditional, lineage-based mode of medical learning – one that has historically followed patrilineage – and say that this emphasis on private master-apprentice instruction does a disservice to the future of Tibetan women, in their potential as healers in general, and in relation to maternal and child health care in particular. However, just as often, particularly in rural areas, one continues to hear refrains such as: *If an amchi comes from a lineage, then his medicine tends to be more powerful or effective.*

In this vein, throughout the TAR and other Tibetan regions of China, one continues to hear stories of lamas who do not practice as professional physicians, but who are known for their production of particular medicines, including healing rituals and protective amulets, or for their expertise as spirit mediums or oracles. There are stories of monks and nuns who live hermits' lives, but whose medicine is renowned; they take few students, if any, and might die with much of the knowledge they possess. One can also visit small, unofficial schools of Tibetan medicine that have cropped up throughout Tibet in which medical instruction is once again married to religious instruction; a few such institutions have even gained access to Tibetan and biomedical medicinal drugs through state-supported village or township clinics and are supported by the local economy through villagers who come to trust in and rely on the monastery for both Tibetan and biomedical treatment. In another vein, some of the more public figures on the Tibetan medicine scene also maintain special relationships with students of unusual talent. In that sense, some of the remnants of lineage-based instruction continue in extracurricular or subtle exchanges within large, state-supported institutions and also across gender lines. Likewise, several famous medical families, such as the inheritors of Khenrab Norbu's medical lineage, maintain private clinics today and continue to take on apprentices. These private modes of instruction, even when carried out in the very public domain of the Barkhor in Lhasa or cities throughout the TAR and other Tibetan areas within the PRC, offer an alternative mode of medical instruction and practice. Here, students gain access not only to oral and written teachings, but also to theoretical knowledge and clinical practice, under the guidance of a teacher and with a smaller group of fellow students than at institutions such as the Tibetan Medical College or the Mentsikhang. Some students might eventually enrol in these large institutions, as a way of receiving further training and state certification. Yet others who have received initial medical instruction from a private teacher might be denied such access to larger institutions, either because they lack the credentials of a formal education – such as examination scores or proficiency in Chinese – or because the methods by which they were taught and the theoretical emphasis of their private teacher varies from that which is considered standard or orthodox medical knowledge within these institutions.

When asked about these shifts in education models and opportunities for today's novice *amchi*, some practitioners will cite the advantages and disadvantages of this shift in emphasis toward institutionalisation and away from less codified or formalised curricula. Some point out that, historically, it was quite common to have one master *amchi* working with a handful of students. Although this model gave students wide access to a variety of Tibetan medical knowledge, both from elder peers and masters, as well as from textual sources, it could also create awkward learning situations, in which a master was trying to speak to people of very different knowledge levels, or would simply speak beyond the knowledge of younger or less experienced students. Today's more institutionalised model has the benefits of a systematic and organised approach to learning and benchmarks for what bodies of knowledge a student should have mastery over when the course is completed. However, in this model of learning, theoretical knowledge and practical, clinical application – both in the realm of diagnosis and treatment and in terms of plant collection and medicine production – are compartmentalised in ways that less formal learning was not. As one elder *amchi* described:

> *Now some amchi are very good with the theory of Tibetan medicine, and even good healers. But although they can prescribe a gar 35 [a Tibetan medicine prescribed for loong imbalances], they don't know how to make it, or sometimes can't identify the ingredients that go into it in their raw form. This is a problem of these new systems of education. It makes it less possible for Tibetan doctors to control the overall quality of their treatment. Before, amchi knew all the elements, even if their knowledge was more limited. They might know very well the plants of their area, for instance, or how to skilfully set a bone, but they might not know much about the subtleties of the three humours. They are two very different kinds of practice, with different results.*

As this perspective illustrates, it is difficult to classify the net effects of these shifts away from private instruction toward institutions as completely positive or negative. And yet, due to the state support for institutionalised learning, the place of Tibetan medicine within the government health care system, and the circumstances under which Tibetan medicines themselves are being made today, the future of private instruction and practice can be considered under threat. However, it is important to note that although the constraints placed on private physicians in the TAR are different from those faced by *amchi* in places like northern Nepal or India, some of the net changes and challenges facing practitioners of *sowa rigpa*, both inside and outside of the PRC, bear a striking resemblance to each other. The forces of rural to urban migration, the decreasing value of vocational practice in exchange for a place in the cash economy, and shifts in educational policy away from learning Tibetan in favour of Chinese, (or English, Hindi, or Nepali) are all impacting the forms, meanings and future of Tibetan medical education. And yet, Tibet differs from these other places in some fundamental respects, namely that there remains an element of – or potential for – more formalised, state-sanctioned suppression of aspects of Tibetan medicine that does not exist in the same way in these other places.

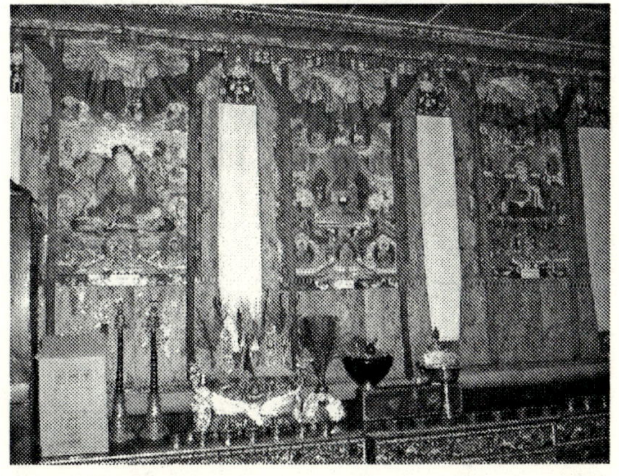

Altar in a medical factory   ©TIN

NGO Funding for Tibetan Medical Education:
A Meeting of Private and Public Spheres

Beyond the state and private practitioners, a third force has begun to transform how one becomes an *amchi*, and what it means to be a Tibetan doctor today. This force is the world of international non-governmental organisations – from small NGOs devoted to particular development arenas such as health or education, to larger, privately funded foundations that support a diversity of projects and programmes. In Tibetan areas of the PRC, such organisations have begun to fund and, in some cases, administer small to medium-sized schools of Tibetan medicine. Again, there is a lot of diversity in this general category of 'NGO': large humanitarian aid organisations; small, private foundations or funds; joint ventures between private and public funds, both within and outside the PRC; and a variety of less formal collaborations that, in certain circumstances, have allowed for interaction between Tibetan exiles and Tibetans who are Chinese citizens. At the time of writing, approximately a dozen international organisations are currently funding projects that support Tibetan medicine within Tibetan areas of the PRC. This support for Tibetan medical education is often in concert with support for hybrid Tibetan and biomedical clinical practice. Given the Chinese state's rather strict stipulations on, and concerns with, the scope of foreign involvement in places like the TAR, as well as the rather straightforward demands for 'local partners' and accountability put forth as part of the language and practical implications of foreign aid, NGOs are often required to work with prefecture-level as well as local (village, township and county) level government bodies. In this respect, the 'private sphere' or 'third space' of NGO funding is – for better or for worse – accountable to, and must operate within, policies, regulations and priorities set forth by various levels of the Chinese state.

This commitment to Tibetan medical education and training (and related areas of support) by NGOs, reveals something of the possibilities and the limitations faced by international organisations working in Tibet today. Namely, although the perpetuation of Tibetan language, culture, and tradition through the path of supporting *sowa rigpa* might be an explicit rational for these organisations' support of Tibetan medicine – the stuff of pretty web pages and shiny brochures aimed at foreign donors – the rationale by which such projects are granted permission to work in Tibet are often more directly tied to discussions of meeting basic health care needs than explicitly encouraging this aspect of Tibetan culture in the PRC today. In other words, foreign aid is often garnered for such endeavours due to the notion that by supporting a Tibetan medical school or clinic, through individual student sponsorship or institutional grants, one is contributing to the survival of Tibetan culture. Yet what it means to support Tibetan survival, particularly in the realm of medicine and health care, remains open to debate and often explicitly ambiguous in the interactions between foreign organisations, donors, and government authorities. In other instances, again paradoxically, although the goals and perspectives of foreign projects might seem to stem from a radically different place than PRC state policies in regard to health care, they can also begin to mirror each other. The power of biomedicine – both in practice and as an ideology about health, well being, and

NGOs Working with Tibetan Medicine in Tibetan areas of the PRC			
Organisation	**Type of Support**	**Areas of Work**	**URL**
Swiss Red Cross	Construction and operating expenses for Tibetan medical school (until fall 2003); follow-up training for graduates from the school	Shigatse Prefecture, TAR	www.redcross.ch/e
Project for Strengthening Traditional Tibetan Medicine (PSTTM)	Direct medical assistance; greenhouses and medicinal plant cultivation; treatment of Big Bone Disease; student scholarships	Lhasa Prefecture, TAR	
Rokpa International	Tibetan medical training programme (based on TMC curriculum); health care centres/clinics; Tibetan medicine production	Chamdo Prefecture, TAR Sichuan Province Qinghai Province Yunnan Province	www.rokpa.org
Trace Foundation	Rural health care training in Tibetan medicine, biomedicine and MCH, as well as health care management; revolving funds for supplying Tibetan medical clinics; funding for advanced training in GMP standardisation	Nagchu and Lhasa Prefectures, TAR Ganzi (Kandze Prefecture), Sichuan Province Hainan Prefecture, Qinghai Province	www.trace.org
American Himalayan Foundation	Scholarship support for Swiss/Tibetan Medical school	Ngari Prefecture, TAR	www.himalayan-foundation.org
Choyin Dorje Traditional Tibetan Medical School/Swiss Tibetan project	Construction, maintenance, and operation of Tibetan medical school and accompanying clinic and small factory	Ngari Prefecture, TAR	
Asia Onlus	Tibetan medical clinic support Tibetan medical education programme support	Hainan Prefecture, Qinghai Province Kanting Prefecture, Sichuan Province	www.asia-onlus.org/
Bridge Fund	Construction and maintenance of clinics using Tibetan medicine and biomedicine	Nagchu and Lhasa Prefectures, TAR Sichuan Province Qinghai Province	http://www.bridgefund.org/
Terma Foundation	Tibetan medicine treatment for childhood illnesses Research on Tibetan medicine	Lhasa and Chamdo Prefectures, TAR	www.terma.org
Tibet Healing Fund	Tibetan medical midwifery and skilled birth attendant training; collaboration with Kumbum Mentsikhang and Qinghai Academy of Tibetan Medicine	Qinghai Province	www.TibetanHealingFund.org
OneHEART	Integrated Tibetan medical and biomedical midwifery, safe motherhood, and neonatal care training	Lhasa Prefecture, TAR	http://www.uuhsc.utah.edu/oneheart/
Seva Foundation	Eye camps; training Tibetan medical doctors in cataracts surgery; workshops on methods to integrate Tibetan and western medicine in health care Programmes	TAR Sichuan Province Qinghai Province	www.seva.org
Tibet Foundation	Integrated Tibetan medical and biomedical maternal and child health and basic health training	Sichuan Province	www.tibet-foundation.org

development articulated by bodies from the Lhasa Health Bureau to the WHO – can come to dominate or usurp the goals of preserving Tibetan culture by supporting Tibetan medicine. The emphasis placed on 'modern science', including a biomedical worldview, as opposed to 'tradition' and the quaint or interesting but still perhaps 'backwards' or 'unscientific' view of *sowa rigpa* is something that surfaces among both international NGO communities and from within PRC government policies, and that can continue to undermine attempts to both support Tibetan medicine and create meaningful and successful programmes in 'integrated' medical education and health care services. This can be the case in more urban, research-oriented projects, as we will discuss in Chapter Four, and it can also come to be in projects founded on models of rural outreach and basic medical training, as well as within both private and public educational institutions.

But what of these NGO-supported schools themselves? What sorts of programmes are funded and how have these interactions between Tibetan, Chinese, and various international players evolved over time? Who are the students at these institutions? The answers are as varied as the donors and local communities in which these endeavours are undertaken, yet we can discern a few themes, the most fundamental of which is the play between tradition and modernity. In addition, we can call attention to the varied forms of knowledge transmission in play at these institutions. From the physical aesthetics of these schools to the structure of the curriculum, many of these schools are an attempt to provide educational opportunities that valorise and adhere to Tibetan culture in general and medical knowledge in particular. The walls of some schools are adorned with sets of the Blue Beryl *thangka* paintings and include prayer rooms and other markers of the relationship between Tibetan medical practice and Tibetan religious practice that are virtually absent from the large, state-supported institutions.

And yet many of these schools and programmes also attempt to prepare students for practicing medicine in rapidly changing social, economic and political contexts – with greater and lesser degrees of success. The students who participate in these programmes tend to be young people in their late teens or early twenties. Most hail from remote areas and have had varying access to primary and secondary education. Some NGOs stipulate that students must come from within the existing health care system: people who are serving as village or township doctors, and who have often had no more than a few years of previous clinical training, but whose basic knowledge of written Tibetan and/or Chinese is good enough to build on. Other students are chosen by quota system from townships and counties, while others still are recruited from local monasteries and nunneries. Sometimes potential students sit for admission exams. The gender split at these small to medium-sized schools tends to reflect both state and foreign priorities of educating girls and women, although some institutions are still primarily devoted to teaching male students. Some schools adhere closely to a five to six year curricula, and are devoted to the study and memorisation of the *Gyushi* and other medical texts, as well as plant identification and pharmacology, basic medicine preparation and clinical apprenticeship. However, schools that are capable of providing all of these opportunities themselves, or who choose to structure their educational programmes along these relatively 'unreformed' lines, are the exception rather than the rule.

More and more schools or educational programmes funded by NGOs are premised on, or have begun to adopt, 'integrated' curricula, in which a more 'classical' course of study based on textual memorisation and hands-on learning under the instruction of a master is altered to reflect the changed access to highly-skilled teachers, the increased presence of and demand for biomedical treatment among Tibetan communities, the developing Tibetan pharmaceutical industry and changing state health care regulations. By 'integrated' we are particularly referring to programmes that attempt to provide a mixture of Tibetan medical and biomedical training. Although there is often more overlap in these smaller institutions between the realms of religious and medical practice, many donors insist on including biomedical training as part of the curriculum. This often takes the form of emergency care, maternal and child health skills or the ability to administer intravenous drugs including antibiotics. While perhaps an intuitive or practical move by foreign projects (often in collaboration with the Chinese state) at one level, the inclusion of biomedical training in the curricula of large and small institutions of Tibetan medicine has further shifted the forms of this education and the future of clinical Tibetan medical practice.

Debates over the inclusion or exclusion of biomedical training in otherwise Tibetan medical curricula relate directly to questions of confidence in and efficacy of Tibetan medicine to which we will return in more detail in Chapter Four. But as most practitioners of any medical system will express, a good healer is one who is grounded in his own medical epistemology, and who has had ample clinical experience in that system of medicine before trying to become skilled in another. Yet schools of Tibetan medicine are experiencing internal pressure, as well as pressure from state and international agencies, to include biomedical techniques and practices in their curricula and to supplement Tibetan medical clinical practice with biomedical training. Part of this shift is dictated by the physical and geographic circumstances in which most *amchi* work and the lack of other health care services in such regions. Another reason for the emphasis on biomedical training comes directly from an acknowledgement of the health care problems that plague many Tibetan communities: high rates of tuberculosis, hepatitis, Sexually Transmitted Diseases (STD) and other communicable diseases for which biomedical treatments can be made readily available. And part of this pressure has everything to do with the power of biomedicine and science: defining paradigms, practices, and belief systems that are far from value-neutral, despite their universalising tendencies.

Reactions among some senior *amchi* who teach at these NGO-funded schools, or even evaluations done by third-party monitors or staff of NGOs themselves, to these calls for 'integrated' curricula in Tibet have been mixed. Some agree with this strategy completely and say that *amchi* should also be trained in biomedical techniques, in order to better serve their communities. Others disagree with this strategy, for both cultural and medical reasons. They suggest instead that biomedical and Tibetan medical practitioners should work in collaboration and that these epistemologies of healing should be allowed to live in two practitioners who can exist side-by-side. Indeed, this has been the model supported by some NGOs.[12] Opponents of such 'integrated' curricula say that these approaches, despite good intentions, embody a naturalised arrogance implicit in many biomedically-driven health care aid projects. They also directly undermine the Tibetan medical training students receive, before this medical knowledge has had a chance to live in the minds and hands of novice practitioners. States and international agencies extol Tibetan medicine as both a 'traditional art' and a 'healing science.' Yet for the sake of – and with the moral force of – saving lives biomedical practices continue to be instituted in ways that can systematically trump Tibetan medical knowledge, practice and medications, or further encourage the biomedicalising of Tibetan medicine. These 'integrated' agendas, in their diverse forms, are directly impacting the choices *amchi* are making, and being forced to make, about the future of their practice, their roles and relations in local contexts.

But the pressures to include or incorporate biomedical practice is not only a result of governmental or non-governmental pressure; it is also a force at play in the interaction between doctors and patients, as well as a reflection of changing expectations and understandings of what medicine is and does, what it means to heal and be healed in the Tibetan context. Some NGO-funded schools have now begun to face the problems created by reproducing a 'traditional' model of education, only to have novice *amchi* return to their communities armed with Tibetan medicines they have only begun to learn how to dispense, without the support of lineage or maturity and experience behind them, and with the added expectations that part of what it means to be a doctor is to know how to administer an IV drip. Some of these novices have therefore stopped practicing medicine in a matter of months, after they have completed an expensive multiple-year program. Others mask their lack of clinical training or inexperience with the sheer power and perceived ease of biomedical treatment, or survive by skipping the diagnostic process altogether, instead prescribing Tibetan or biomedical treatments based on cursory case histories and superficial examination of symptoms. In some instances, NGOs are working with local communities and health care authorities to create additional clinical training programmes at county hospitals practicing Tibetan and biomedicine, and in some instances at the Mentsikhang in Lhasa or branch clinics.

In addition to the problem of having access to good quality teachers and enough clinical experience during the course of a novice *amchi*'s education to make developing a career as a Tibetan doctor viable and finding a place in the health care system, either as a state employee or a private practitioner, the other huge challenge facing students who graduate from these institutions is the medicine itself: who has access to it, who makes it, how much it costs and whether or not it 'works' – all topics to be explored in the next two chapters.

12 Trace Foundation, for instance, has developed a model of 'Two Systems, One Roof' in which practitioners of Tibetan medicine work alongside health care workers trained in general biomedical practice and maternal and child health.

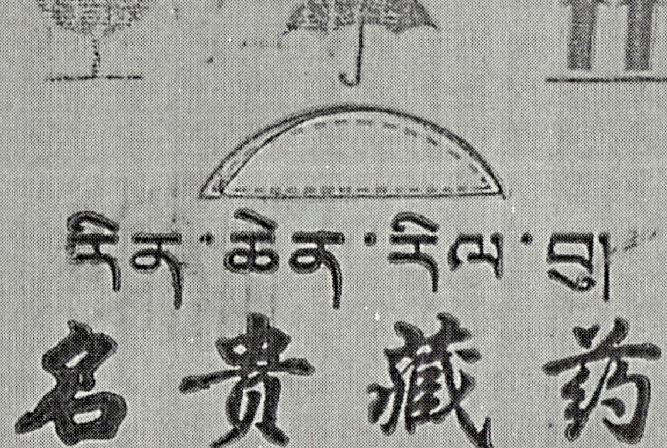

Rinchen Ripu box ©TIN

Chapter Three

From the *Gyushi* to GMP: Production, Standardisation and Commercialisation

Yuthog Lam, a glittery thoroughfare in downtown Lhasa, links the Barkhor market area and Jokhang temple to the central administrative complex of the TAR government. Literally and figuratively, this street connects old and new Tibet. Polished stone slabs pave the sidewalk. Plastic palm trees in day-glo colours, fountains spurting rainbows of water and oversized mushroom-shaped seats that, when sat upon, play the latest Chinese and Tibetan pop tunes, further create an Oxford Circus-meets-Las Vegas aesthetic. Department stores, electronics outlets and Beijing boutiques stand out among the commercial shops that line this road. In the winter, when Lhasa is inundated with pilgrims from Kham and Amdo, Nagchu and Ngari, one can watch nomad women peruse the displays of electric rice cookers and stare in wonder and amazement at the escalators. In spring and summer, Lhasa teenagers, Chinese and Tibetan alike, enliven the street as they loiter, waiting to be seen. Fresh flowers bloom in porcelain planters and

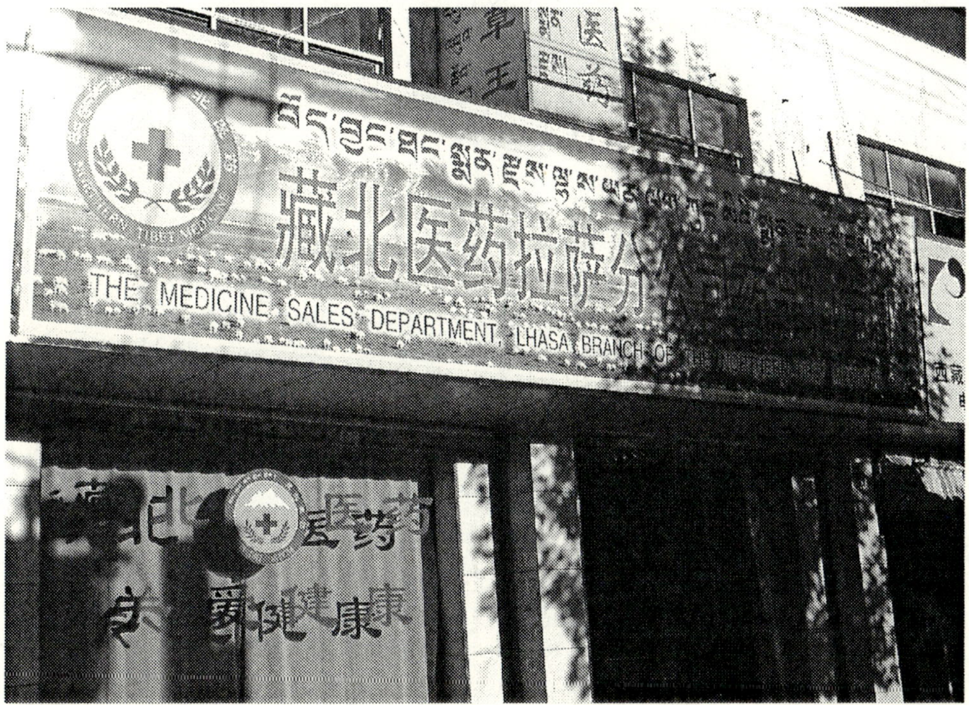

Medicine shop in Lhasa ©TIN

the rickshaws come streaming by. At one end of the street rests a rebuilt Yuthog Bridge – another marker of old Tibet's social geography, which once linked the Potala palace complex with the old city of Lhasa, now dwarfed by the scale of Lhasa's modern-day expansion. Near the top of the street sits the out-patient Mentsikhang, still a centre of Lhasa life, though now masked somewhat by the gold jewellery salesmen and endless kiosks of cheap denim, incense and multi-collared *kathag*, Tibetan offering scarves, that line this section of the road.

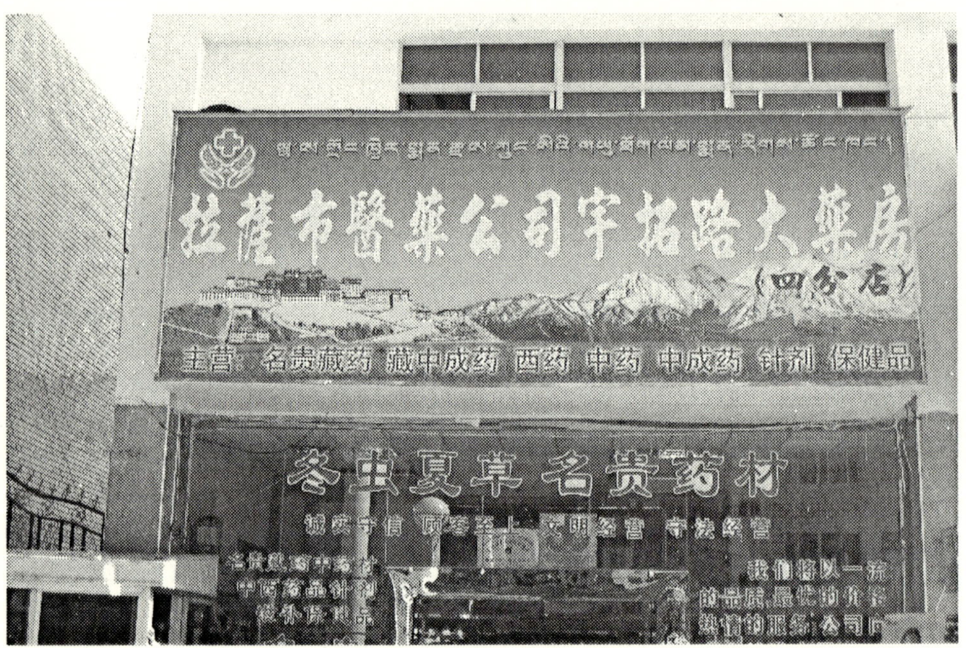

Yuthog Lam   ©TIN

But the most striking thing about Yuthog Lam is the number of stores devoted to selling Tibetan medicine. In the space of two long city blocks, one encounters no less than a dozen such stores, all advertising various brands of Tibetan medicines. Some are devoted entirely to the sale of ready-made Tibetan pills and powders while others are hybrid designer pharmacies, selling both Tibetan and biomedical remedies, from Valium to *ratna sampel*, a kind of Tibetan medicine pill. Some stores offer displays of exotic raw materials: gift packages of saffron, snakeskin, and *yartsa gunbu*, [see Text Box], tied up with red and gold ribbons; glass jars filled with dried mushrooms, ginseng and a decidedly Sino-Tibetan cornucopia of aphrodisiacs and tonics. Others still are combination pharmacies and souvenir outlets where consumers can buy fake yak heads, Khampa-style knives and miniature reproductions of the Potala palace, along with made for export 'precious pills' (*rinchen rilbu*).

If the key to successful tourist consumerism is to fashion the stereotyped 'essence' of a culture or a place and make it available for purchase, then there is no greater symbol of the present and future of Tibet than this market for Tibetan medicinals. (It is also interesting to note that most shoppers on Yuthog Lam are mainland Chinese, not foreign tourists.) What is advertised for sale here is nothing less than Tibet itself; its cultural and scientific heritage, its ecological resources and its place in outsiders' imaginations as a heavenly realm, capable of producing miraculous cures and the elixirs of enlightenment. But these prominent storefront displays also illustrate, by omission, the more overarching effects of this drive to standardise and capitalise on Tibetan medicines. Namely, they point to the dwindling number of amchi who have the time, knowledge or resources to make their own medicines. They hint at the national and international trade in medicinal ingredients and corresponding depletion of Tibet's flora and fauna in order to keep up with market demand. The Tibetan pharmaceutical industry also does its best to mask the cultural, political and economic pressures placed on medicine factories to modernize their production methods – to depart from traditional techniques or face closure in the coming years. The fancy storefronts and pretty packages deflect attention away from the rising costs and, some argue, decreasing efficacy of the medicines themselves, as well as the threat of decreasing access of rural Tibetans to good quality, affordable Tibetan medicines.

This chapter is an exploration into the forces at play in these changes. It is an attempt to account for the growing commercial investments in Tibetan medicines and the pressures to standardise Tibetan pharmaceuticals. In addition to debates about efficacy, these pressures arise both from within and outside circles of Tibetan medical practice and are impacting *sowa rigpa* practice, as we shall explore in more detail in Chapter Four. One hears stories of what is sometimes referred to as a 'Tibetan medical mafia' in which corruption and huge money making schemes dominate, and where producing quality medicines is a low priority. The reality of medicine production and sale in Tibet today is further complicated by the growing interest in clinical research of Tibetan medicine in China and the west, as we will discuss more in Chapter Four, as well as the manufacturing, standardisation, licensing, and drug registration policies that are being implemented in pharmaceutical factories throughout the PRC.

It is also interesting to note that the Tibetan medicine industry not only ties Tibet to the rest of China through capital investments and markets, but also ironically enforces a vision of what greater Tibet is that includes parts of Sichuan, Gansu, Yunnan and Qinghai provinces – areas that correspond closely to the geopolitical borders of Tibet at very different points in history, not only from the period immediately preceding the Chinese 'liberation' but also shadowing older borders and trade routes. It is a sense of Tibetan domain defined by ecology – and the potential to capitalise on nature – more than politics, but one that has political connotations nonetheless. In addition, this trade in *materia medica* and ready-made medicines is also part of the larger global phenomenon of 'alternative medicine' markets, and that includes connections between Tibetans living in China and Tibetan exile communities.

What is yartsa gunbu?

Translated as 'summer grass winter insect', *yartsa gunbu* is the Tibetan name for the product of a singular ecological symbiosis between a caterpillar and a mushroom. The tiger moth lays its eggs on grasses and the larvae emerge during the early summer. Synchronously, a parasitic fungus (L. *Cordyceps sinensis*), found between 13,000 and 16,000 feet in Tibet, India, Bhutan and Nepal, releases its spores, which are then transported by the wind. Through chance and the profligate nature of fungi, the spores land on the caterpillar's body and bore up through its head, giving *yartsa gunbu* its unique centaur-like appearance of being both a grass and an insect. Once it is harvested, *yartsa gunbu* is dried, ground up and mixed with liquid – often water or distilled hard alcohol – to make a powerful tonic said to increase one's vigour, endurance and libido. Tibetan doctors also say that *yartsa gunbu* helps improve kidney function and circulation.

The market for *yartsa gunbu* throughout Tibet and the Himalayas is booming. In highland Nepal, one kilogram of *yartsa gunbu* (whose collection was recently made legal by the Government of Nepal) fetches more than NRS.100,000 (approx: £730; €1,050; $1,350; 11,130 RMB). In Lhasa, the price for a kilogram of *yartsa gunbu* ranges from 10,000 to more than 30,000 RMB (approx: £650-£1,960; €950-€2850; $1,200-$3,600), depending on the quality. Throughout the Tibetan Plateau, the trade and sale in *yartsa gunbu* is thriving, with many highland pastures in the TAR, as well as in Kham and Amdo, boasting the presence of these medicinal creatures. The market for *yartsa gunbu* remains focused on export to other parts of the PRC as well as Taiwan. Many rural Tibetans hope to make small fortunes through the collection and sale of this unique medicinal. Indeed, some *amchi* rely on an annual sale of *yartsa gunbu* to fund the purchase of medicinal ingredients or ready-made medicines. **(See TIN's Tibet 2002: A Yearbook: Page 21 *Testimony on yartsa gunbu* collection in Tibet.)**

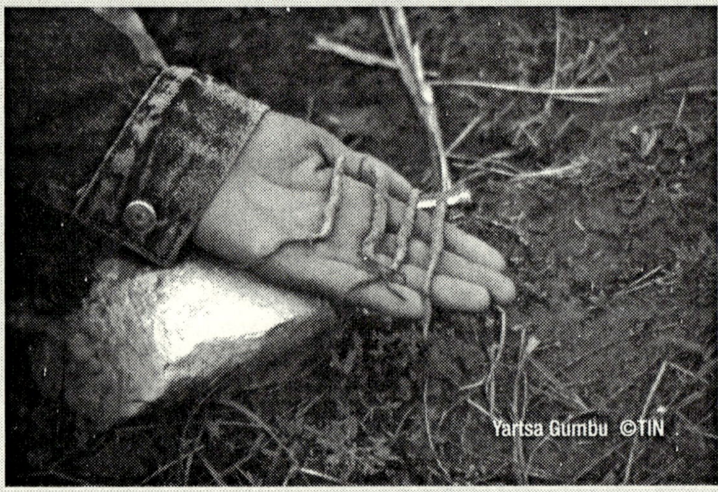

Materia Medica: Pharmacology, Trade, Depletion, Conservation, and Cultivation

In order to appreciate the extent to which Tibetan medicines themselves are changing, as a result of commercialisation and standardization, let us begin with the plants, stones, soils and animal products that make up Tibetan medicines and take a closer look at Tibetan pharmacology.

The *Gyushi* states that all substances on earth carry medicinal value. Tibetan pharmacology draws a connection between the human body and the natural environment, as well as guidelines for the collection of medicinal plants that can be deemed environmentally friendly, at least in theory. The fundamental tenets of Tibetan pharmacology are an extension of the theory of the five elements, in relation to the three humours. Beyond this, pharmacology can be understood in traditional Tibetan medicine as following the Seven Limb Procedure as outlined in the *Gyushi* for identifying, collecting, cultivating and processing plant and other ingredients into medicines. It is worthwhile listing the main points of these seven limbs in order to see just how much the circumstances under which Tibetan medicines are being made in China today depart from these edicts, at least in the context of large-scale medical factories.[13]

The First Limb of this procedure discusses the growth of medicinal plants in their natural habitat. Places where medicinal plants grow should be fertile and devoid of environmental destruction, pollution, contamination from poisonous animals, hail or fire. Beyond this, medicines with cooling power should be harvested from high and cold areas, while the reverse is true for those ingredients with heating properties. (Remember from the outline of Tibetan medicine presented in Chapter One that *sowa rigpa*, like Ayurveda, classifies medicinal ingredients as well as the humours as either 'hot' or 'cold' in nature.) Adhering to these principles helps ensure the efficacy of the medicines, as does harvesting plants of superior quality. The Second Limb of the procedure instructs amchi and other harvesters in the time that medicines should be collected. The instructions for harvesting and collection in this section link the five elements and

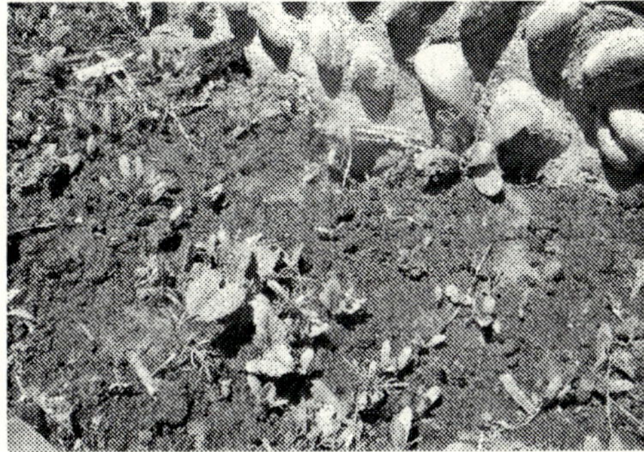

Chumdsa cultivation   ©TIN

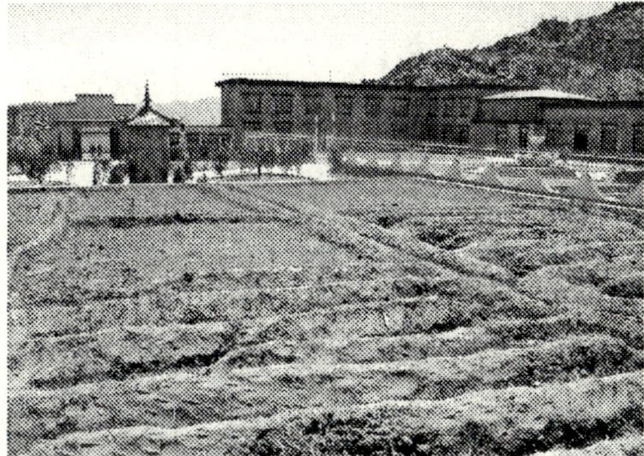

Shongbala cultivation   ©TIN

13 Outline of Seven Limb Procedures adapted from Men-tsee-khang (2001: 67-70).

three humours not only to botanical properties but also to phenology and to the specific kinds of illnesses and imbalances that each kind of ingredient helps treat. For example, this limb instructs: *leaves, rubber plants and shoots pacify diseases of the six hollow organs, bone marrow, and spongy bone. They are collected during summer, i.e. the sixth month of the Tibetan year, when plants grow fully.* This limb also gives detailed instruction on medicinal ingredient collection in relation to the cycles of the moon (e.g. during the waxing of the moon, the potency of medicinal plants increases) and astrological calculations. Furthermore, it instructs the physician-harvester to collect with right motivation and lists *mantra* that should be recited during collection to help increase the plants' potencies. The Third Limb refers to the removal of toxic impurities from medicinal ingredients and instructs on how ingredients should be washed, separated

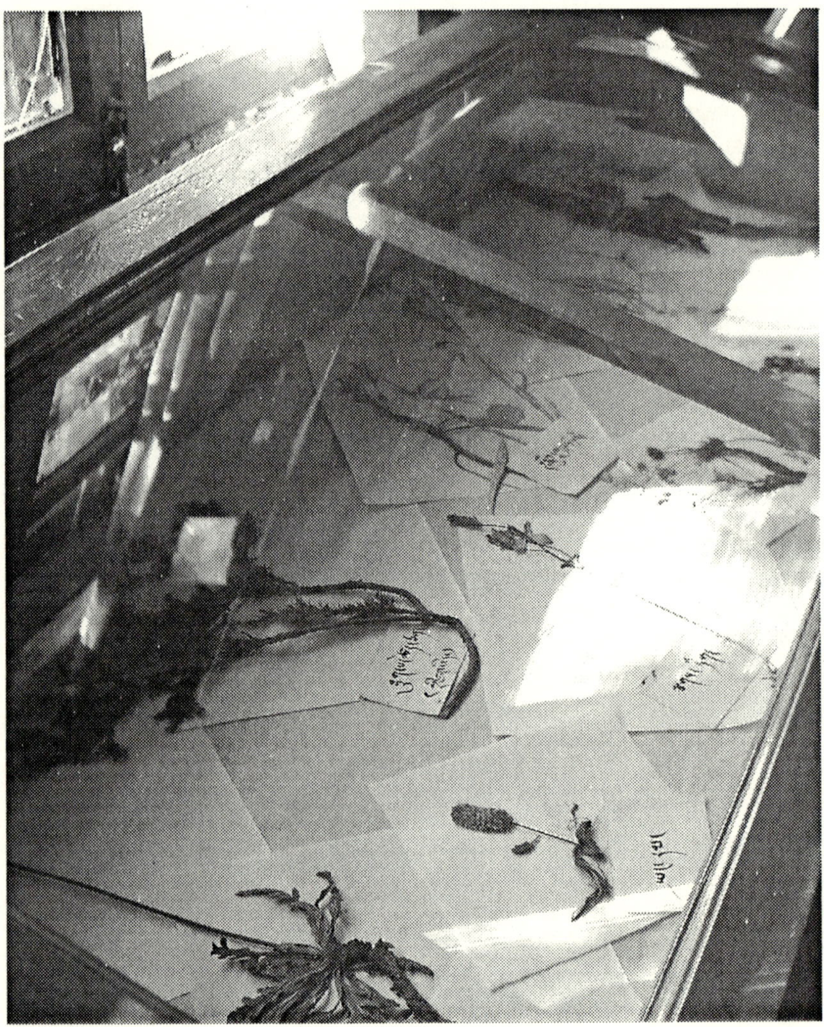

Ingredients display   ©TIN

and refined. The Fourth Limb is concerned with how medicinal plants should be dried. It instructs: *cooling powered medicines are dried in shady and airy areas, while warm powered medicines are dried in the sun and near fire.* Furthermore, this limb states that each type of medicinal plant should be kept separate at this stage to prevent contamination. The Fifth Limb is an edict on maintaining efficacy, stating that all plant medicines should be used while they are fresh, within twelve months of collection. However, this varies substantially for medicinal ingredients derived from earth, mineral or animal products. The Sixth Limb is basically a more subtle exegesis on toxicology and pharmacology, describing how particular kinds of ingredients can be combined to increase effectiveness and decrease potential side effects. The Seventh Limb describes suitable combinations of medicinal ingredients and the compounding process. This final limb goes into the most detail on the kinds of medicinal ingredients used in Tibetan pharmacology, namely gems (*rinpoche*), stones (*do*), soils (*sa*), mucilaginous substances (*tsi*), shrubs (*thang*), herbs (*ngo*) and animal products (*sog chag*). It also details the various forms that medicines can take and instructs on their preparations. These include not only the classic Tibetan medical pill, or rilbu, but also decoctions, powders, medicinal pastes, medicinal butter, wine, ash, highly concentrated decoctions, herbal compounds and gem compounds.

Tibetan *materia medica* is also a perfect illustration of the larger dynamic within Tibetan culture between the value of things or ideas that originate outside Tibet and those that are classified as internal or intrinsic. In Tibetan, the phrase *chi – nang* literally means 'outside – inside.' This can be used to describe social, political and geographic differences, such as the boundaries of historical or present-day Tibet, or distinguishing non-Buddhists from Buddhists in the Tibetan context. In connection to medicinal ingredients, though, this distinction between those that come from outside Tibet and things that are indigenous also relate directly to the power and potency of medicines themselves. Within Tibetan *pharmacopoeia*, much that is valued is imported. Perhaps the most striking example of this is a ru, the seed from a tree of Indian origin (L. *chebulic myrobalan* or *Terminalia chebula Retz.*) that is held in the hands of the Medicine Buddha. It, like other things that come from outside Tibet – including Buddhism – has been incorporated into the essence of what it means for a person, or a practice, or a medicine to be Tibetan. Some of the key ingredients in Tibetan medicines come from the Indian subcontinent or low, hot areas of the PRC. As such, an active and thriving trade in medicinal plants and other ingredients is a premise on which Tibetan medicine has been based for centuries – even among amchi practicing in what are today extremely remote communities. This trade not only

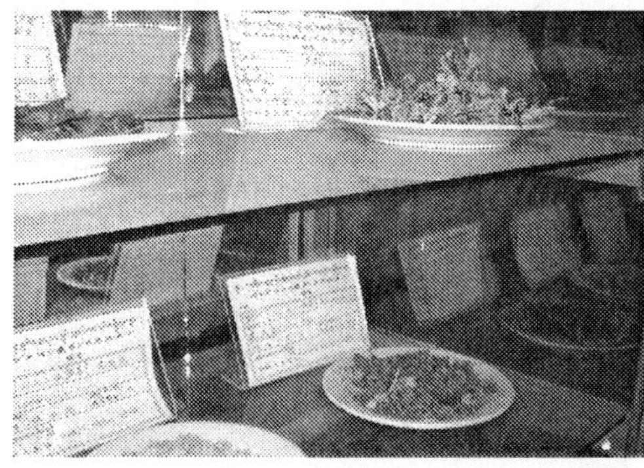

Medicinal ingredients   ©TIN

includes botanical ingredients but also

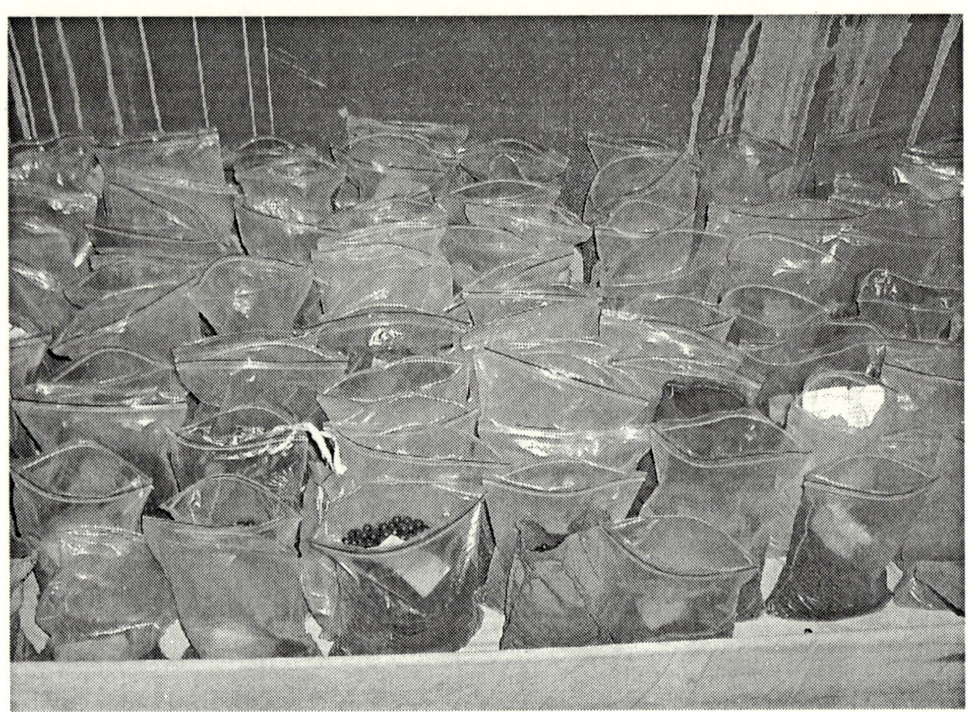

Homemade pills   ©TIN

precious and semi-precious stones, as well as animal products such as rhinoceros horns or crab shells. In this sense, part of the creativity and power of Tibetan medicine comes from its ability to not only transform poison into medicine and to value the medicinal properties in every substance, but also it its ability to use and incorporate so many influences and substances that originate outside the Land of Snows.

But how has this pharmacology changed today? How have pressures, from species extinction and global biodiversity legislation to geopolitics, through which a contiguous landscape is divided up into nation-states, changed Tibetan doctors' access to the ingredients on which their medicine is based? It is common to hear Tibetan doctors, particularly those practicing in rural Tibetan communities, complain about the decreasing kinds, quantity and quality of medicinal plants. They recognise that this depletion is due in part to over-harvesting for commercial use – a problem that is not unique to the TAR or other Tibetan areas of the PRC, but that has played out in this national context in particular ways. This depletion and decrease in quality of plants is also tied directly to other forms of environmental degradation, from deforestation, mining, overgrazing or the use of chemical fertilizers or poisons on agricultural fields and rangelands, to urban pollution and larger climatic shifts from global warming. And, in the context of modern Tibet, environmental degradation has also been discursively linked directly to the *karma* of political oppression, as well as the net effects of 'development' and economic liberalization on the land. Many Tibetans, particularly those in rural areas, feel that control over their lives and landscape has been wrested from them, concentrated instead in the hands of politicians and business people, who may be ethnically Han Chinese or Chinese Muslims (Hui) or Tibetan. All of these forces are profoundly affecting the ecology of the Tibetan Plateau; the production, consumption and commodification of Tibetan medicine bears directly on the health of Tibetan ecology as well as on the health and access to health care of Tibetan people.

Throughout Tibetan areas of the PRC today, the rise in capital investments and the creation of a major for-profit industry around products that require rare or even endangered natural resources, some from marginal and sensitive high-mountain ecologies, means that conceiving of Tibetan medicine as big business is inherently unsustainable. The growing industry of Tibetan pharmaceuticals has meant the rise in demand for medicinal ingredients, the creation of labour markets for collection in rural communities and the purchase of *materia medica* by large factories that are unconcerned with the principles outlined in the Seven Limb Procedure of the *Gyushi*. Instead, the model of collection most often follows market rules of supply and demand and does not pay attention to the state of mind of those collecting, the quality (including the taste and smell) of each plant, or with purity or quality of medicinal specimens. Many rural Tibetans, desperate for cash in an increasingly monetised economy, also collect medicinal ingredients for sale to large factories or middlemen. In the summertime in particular, it is not uncommon to see dozens of villagers out collecting from valleys or hillsides, or to see large lorries roll into townships, ready to purchase in bulk ingredients for wholesale prices. These herbal ingredients are then bought up, primarily by large state or privately owned factories, and mass-produced into Tibetan formulas.

The big business of Tibetan medicine inside the PRC provides a very interesting contrast to the narratives – and, to a certain extent, the realities – of conservation and biological diversity, as well as control over the trade in medicinal plants by national governments, international agencies, global conventions and local 'user groups' that proliferate in the South Asian context and that bear directly on amchi practicing in Nepal, India and Bhutan.[14] In Tibet, given the proportionally greater number of Tibetan medical factories and the higher profit margins, few individuals or organizations are working on issues of sustainable harvesting of medicinal plants. At this time, there are reported to be fewer experiments in medicinal plant cultivation in Tibetan areas of the PRC than in India and Nepal, for instance.

Yet, in recognition of these environmental and ecological concerns, some governmental and non-governmental organizations have begun both large and small-scale cultivation experiments. The Technology and Commerce Bureau of the TAR government and the

14 In Nepal, India, and Bhutan, both international and regional or local NGOs, as well as governments, are very active in the planning and execution of conservation-oriented legislation and joint conservation and development initiatives. The World Wildlife Fund for Nature, and its branches in all three of these South Asian countries, have been leaders in this respect, as have branches of Conservation International, and the Medicinal and Aromatic Plant Programme in Asia (MAPPA). The Convention on International Trade in Endangered Species (CITES) also bears on the use and collection of medicinal ingredients, both by commercial harvesters or poachers and by *amchi* and other ethnomedical healers, in these countries, as does national park legislation. Still, depletion at the hands of commercial interests and *amchi* themselves continues to threaten the future of Tibetan medicine production and practice.

Tibet Academy of Agricultural and Animal Sciences (TAAAS), as well as the Mentsikhang and a few private factories, have begun to invest in the trial cultivation of selected medicinal plants. Government monies have allocated for greenhouses and large and small-scale experiments are underway throughout the TAR, particularly in Kongpo and areas around Lhasa, as well as in other parts of the Tibetan Plateau that fall outside the TAR borders. For instance, the Mentsikhang factory is now conducting cultivation trials on special and rare medicinal plants on 300 square metres of land on the edges of urban Lhasa. Likewise, these areas are also beginning to see an increase in grassroots organising around issues of environmental degradation. At least two foreign NGOs working within the TAR are now supporting greenhouses and cultivation experiments for medicinal plants, as well as educating villagers about sustainable harvesting methods. Despite such efforts, it remains difficult to convince Tibetan villagers that selling off their local resources to representatives of large-scale factories, while bringing short-term benefits, is harming the long-term health of both their environment and themselves.

When asked about this issue of sustainable collection and medicinal plant cultivation, Tibetan amchi working at state or private factories, and Tibetan medical industry representatives alike, often responded by saying that Tibet (and China) is vast and rich in resources, and that, with the exception of certain ingredients derived from endangered species (such as Tibetan antelope horns), ingredients are plentiful. Others are inherently sceptical about cultivation; they say plants are more potent when collected from the wild, and doubt the ability of certain plants to grow under cultivated conditions. Undoubtedly, there are cultural and biological truths to these assertions, but they also beg the question of sustainability and the future of Tibetan medicines not only as high-priced export commodities but also as locally available treatments.

Let us now turn toward the circumstances under which Tibetan medicines are being manufactured, particularly in the large state and private factories.

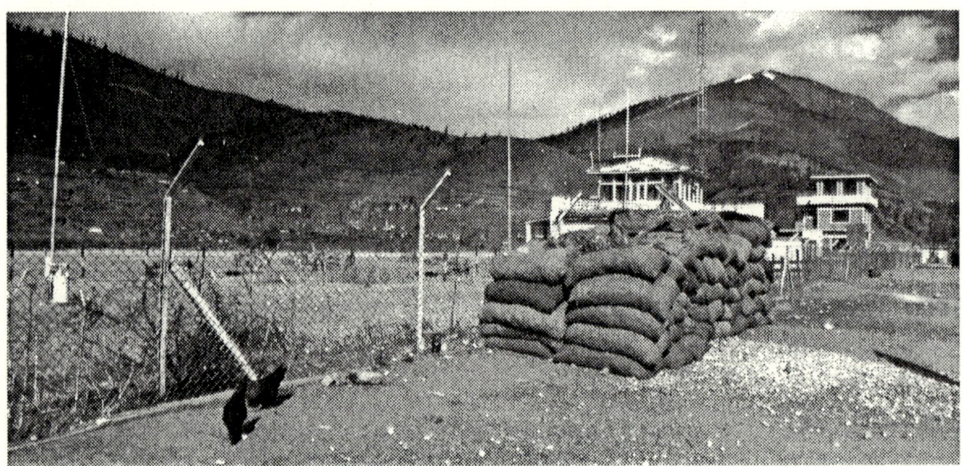

Medical plants shipped to Tibet, Jumla, West nepal   ©TIN

Medical Factories, Good Manufacturing Practices, and Tibetan Drug Registration

Good Manufacturing Practices (GMP) standards are international standards based on documents issued by the World Health Organisation (WHO) about the standardisation of ingredients and the hygienic preparation of medicines. The GMP standards are interpreted and implemented on a national level, they do not just apply to Tibetan medicine, but are enforced worldwide, and in the PRC are applied to the production of Traditional Chinese Medicines and biomedical factories as well.[15] The specific guidelines, which have been established in relation to Tibetan medicine, focus mainly on cleaning, drying and compounding techniques, as well as the removal of poisons from medicinal ingredients. These GMP standards have been particularly important in relation to the production of *rinchen rilbu*, the Tibetan 'Precious Pills' that are not only the hottest medicinal commodity both for internal and export markets, but that also traditionally contain many potent active ingredients e.g. purified and detoxified heavy metals, including lead and mercury.

So far, the implementation of GMP on Tibetan medicine appears to have been rather one-sided. Whereas GMP is a flexible framework, which can accommodate various medical practices, and incorporate, for example, anthroposophic medicine or homoeopathy without distortions, there has been no similar attempt in the PRC to create specific GMP-regulation for Tibetan medicine, i.e. to formulate the regulations in a way that would protect and safeguard manufacturing of Tibetan herbal medicine. Rather, GMP is generally interpreted as a sort of superficial and fuzzy 'modernisation', which appears to aim at quick marketability instead of thoughtful and sustainable adaptation to modern standards of hygiene.

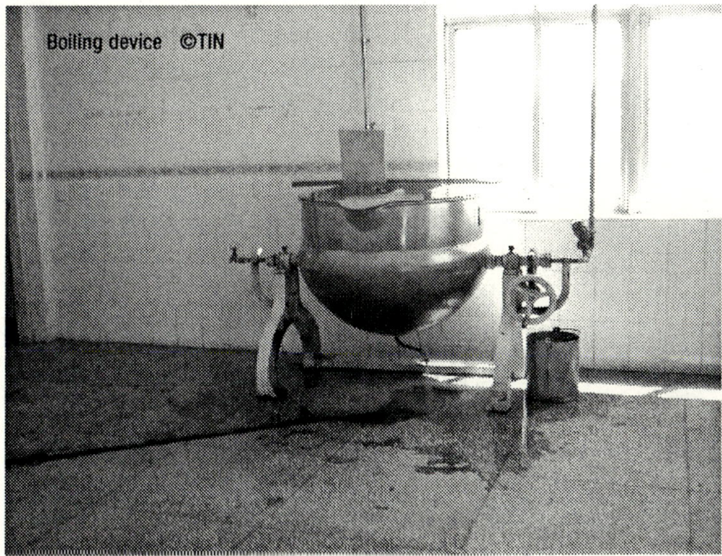

15 It should be remarked, though, that Chinese medical products have a low credibility in the west, since the Chinese authorities are believed to be rather lax in implementing GMP. In western countries it is strictly forbidden to produce medicine outside the GMP-framework.

Poisons in Tibetan Medicine?

Some of the rinchen rilbu varieties of Tibetan medicine as well as other kinds of compounds contain very potent ingredients, among them heavy metals and other elements that must be purified or detoxified before they can be used in final preparations of medications. Many of the *rinchen rilbu* varieties of Tibetan medicine as well as other kinds of compounds contain heavy metals and other elements that must be purified or detoxified before they can be used in final preparations of medications. This is particularly true of medicines that contain mercury. Although these detoxification techniques have been used for centuries, the presence of such ingredients in Tibetan medicines has caused significant alarms among international individuals and organisations that are otherwise interested in the export and clinical use of Tibetan medicine in the west. In response to these concerns, some producers of Tibetan medicine for export have decided to exclude these ingredients from the medicines altogether; others have tried to ensure that the medicines are prepared in accordance with Tibetan medical recipes, and at the same time meet standardisation and toxicity testing requirements.

Pilot projects have been established in relation to this issue, particularly the use of mercury. There are preliminary results from one such project currently underway among patients at the Men-tsee-khang in Dharamsala. So far, this study has revealed that while the particular medicine in question contained more than 40% mercury, primarily in the form of mercuric sulphide, blood and urine tests on patients reveal no mercury and no signs of its toxicity. This and other research suggests that the process by which mercury is detoxified, according to Tibetan pharmacology and then used in compound medicines, creates a situation in which the mercury bonds with proteins and other enzymes and facilitates a non-toxic interaction with positive therapeutic effects. (Sallon, et al 2003) However, these results remain partly controversial and further research remains to be done.

The application of GMP standards by the PRC government to Tibetan medicines has translated into the need to create new and special factories and invest in machines for production and packaging of medicines. Interestingly, although GMP standard regulations do not insist that factories invest in the most expensive and high-tech methods of production – but rather legislate general rules about manufacturing circumstances, hygiene and standardisation – most large factories engage in a kind of competition with each other to see who can build the biggest, most expensive factories and garner the most capital investment. But this combined need and desire to invest in new buildings and the latest technology has also meant that previously self-sustaining and smaller-scale Tibetan medical factories are in the market for investors; mainland and overseas Chinese now own majority shares in many Tibetan medical factories. In addition, these enterprises are, by necessity or desire, turning away from the primary purpose of making good quality medicines as defined by the *Gyushi* and other texts, as well as generations of *sowa rigpa* practitioners, and toward making medicines which formally follow GMP standards without even trying to adapt these within the specific context of *sowa rigpa* and are often geared for markets outside Tibet.

That being said, today many of the large Tibetan medical factories also continue non-GMP standard production of medicines geared toward non-commercial purposes. For instance, of the more than 350 kinds of medicines produced at the Mentsikhang factory in Lhasa, only forty-odd medicines are currently produced to GMP standards and marketed as such. The rest of the medicines are made in a more 'traditional' style, although the quality of the ingredients going into these medicines remains an issue, as we shall explore in more detail below. These are the medicines that eventually supply not only the in-patient and out-patient Mentsikhang hospitals in Lhasa, but also branch hospitals and clinics throughout the TAR, as well as most county hospitals and township clinics.

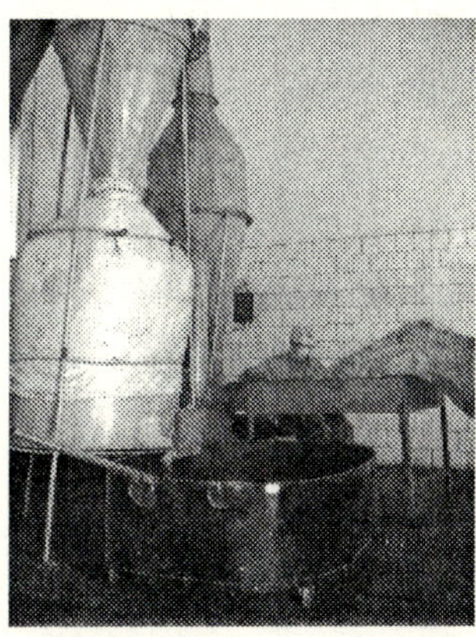

Grinding device   ©TIN

These non-GMP medicines are technically illegal to sell commercially, but they remain readily available in urban areas and are still relatively inexpensive, though prices have risen over the past decade. The divide that is created between GMP and non-GMP medicines, both in terms of its impact on clinical practice and in terms of Tibetan medicine distribution to and use in rural areas, will be discussed in more detail in the following chapter. In interviews with Tibetan doctors and medicine factory executives, it has been mentioned that by 2005, all Tibetan medical production will have to confirm to GMP regulations. If enforced, and without attempts to harmonize 'traditional' medical practice and international medical standards, such a policy could have drastic effects on the accessibility, quality and price of Tibetan medicines for Tibetan patients.[16]

In addition to the issues surrounding the introduction of new standards of medicinal practice, drug registration for Tibetan pharmaceuticals is also impacting production, sales, and distribution methods. While GMP policies refer to the conditions of drug manufacturing and issues of quality and standardization in this respect, the TAR Drug Registration Department is in charge of overseeing clinical tests on Tibetan medicines and ensuring that the efficacy of the medicines are established in chemical and clinical terms before licenses are issued for the commercial production and sale of these medicines. Before 2000, when the TAR Drug Registration Department was first established, and Good Clinical Practices (GCP) introduced, the protocols surrounding registering Tibetan drugs in the PRC were nascent; today, all Tibetan medicines

---

16 International standards of medicine production, like GMP and Tibetan medicine, do not need to be viewed as incompatible per se. Experience outside the PRC and in western countries show that, with a sound knowledge of both, acceptable *modi vivendi* can be found, and almost all difficulties bound to the adaptation of such different medical standards can be overcome. This, however, requires an intensive, careful and thoughtful process, the need of which does not seem to have been acknowledged so far in the PRC.

produced for commercial sale must conform to the same standards of clinical testing as Traditional Chinese Medicines and biomedicines produced in the PRC. Drug registration numbers (i.e. the authorisations required to market the drugs) are only issued for Tibetan medicines once they have gone through a three-stage protocol, involving chemical analyses, animal testing and finally, clinical testing on human populations – a process that is often very costly and that has only been undertaken by the largest Tibetan pharmaceutical factories. However, the issuance of new drug registration numbers, as well as the monitoring and enforcement of drug registration protocols, varies between the TAR and other regions of the PRC that produce Tibetan medicines (e.g. Kham and Amdo). The issue of drug registration is still only a primary concern for the largest Tibetan medical factories, not the small to medium-sized private factories, which are often connected to clinics.

Before moving on to a discussion of private medicine production, let us take a closer look at the Lhasa Mentsikhang factory, as an example of the effects of standardisation and commercial demands on Tibetan medicine today. The factory was built in 1964, and has been steadily expanding. It was made to conform to Chinese GMP policies in 1996, and has continued to modernise its methods of production, as well as invest in its sales and marketing departments, in the last decade. The factory boasts annual sales of approximately 30 million RMB (approx: £1,960,918; €2,931,714; $3,624,386), produces more than 400 tons of medicine annually and is the largest Tibetan pharmaceutical factory in the TAR. As an English translation of the 'General Description of History and Activities' of the Mentsikhang Tibetan Medical Factory puts it:

> *Now the Factory produces a variety of products: over 350 kinds of drugs, 52 of which have been granted official PRC drug registration numbers. Among these, 13 kinds of product have been approved by Ministry of Health as 'national protected traditional medicines,' and 15 of these products are listed as 'basic drugs' of the state. These kinds of Tibetan medicines, designated as 'sweet dew', are beneficial for treating cardiovascular, digestive and other diseases; they are also beneficial for alleviating other physical problems.*

As this quote serves to illustrate, the Mentsikhang and other GMP-standard arms of private Tibetan medical factories are not, for the most part, investing in cheap, good quality medicines for use by rural doctors. Rather, they are focused on producing 'designer' Tibetan medicines and new products, such as medicated plasters and vitality-boosting capsules, for urban Tibetan, Chinese and export markets – the merchandise filling the shelves of Yuthog Lam stores. Ironically, the implementation of new international standards has not led to a full acknowledgement of Tibetan medicine, since due to regulations such as those of the US Food and Drug Administration (FDA), Tibetan medicines must not be called 'medicine' when they are exported, but are instead called 'nutritional/food/dietary supplements' – a reality that further complicates the global implications of Tibet's stake in medicine markets.[17]

17 Similar problems exist with Traditional Chinese Medicine (TCM) and its use in western countries. It should be remarked that TCM, though labeled as 'traditional', is in fact a modernised or even sanitised version of ancient Chinese Medicine. TCM has been adapted to the needs and demands of a modern, global society.

Profile of a Factory: The Cheezheng Group (Qizheng) and the Nyingchi Qizheng Tibetan Pharmaceutical Factory

The Cheezheng Group and the Nyingchi Qizheng Tibetan Pharmaceuticals Factory is one of the most successful private producers of Tibetan medicinal products in the PRC. Based in Nyingchi County in Kongpo, the site of the Namyi Gully, where India's Assam plain and the Qinghai-Tibet Plateau meet, its reputation as a producer of high quality, (and GMP-quality), medicines has much to do with their choice of location in the lush Kongpo region, as well as their satellite suppliers and producers in Gansu Province. Nyingchi County is known as a "natural medicine storehouse" and its ecology hosts more than 1000 varieties of medicinal plants. According to the company's literature, the company has aimed "to exploit and make use of these medicinal resources, and develop Nyingchi's economy with local characteristics." The Cheezheng Group, set up on August 18, 1993, is a non-governmental hi-tech enterprise that plans to inherit and develop traditional Tibetan medicine. It owns a 667-hectare medicinal herbs protected area in the Yarlung Zangbo River area, and seems invested in both cultivation experiments and conservation efforts, particularly of rare high altitude species. The Cheezheng Group has two GMP-standard Tibetan medicine factories in Nyingchi in the TAR and Gannan in Gansu Province

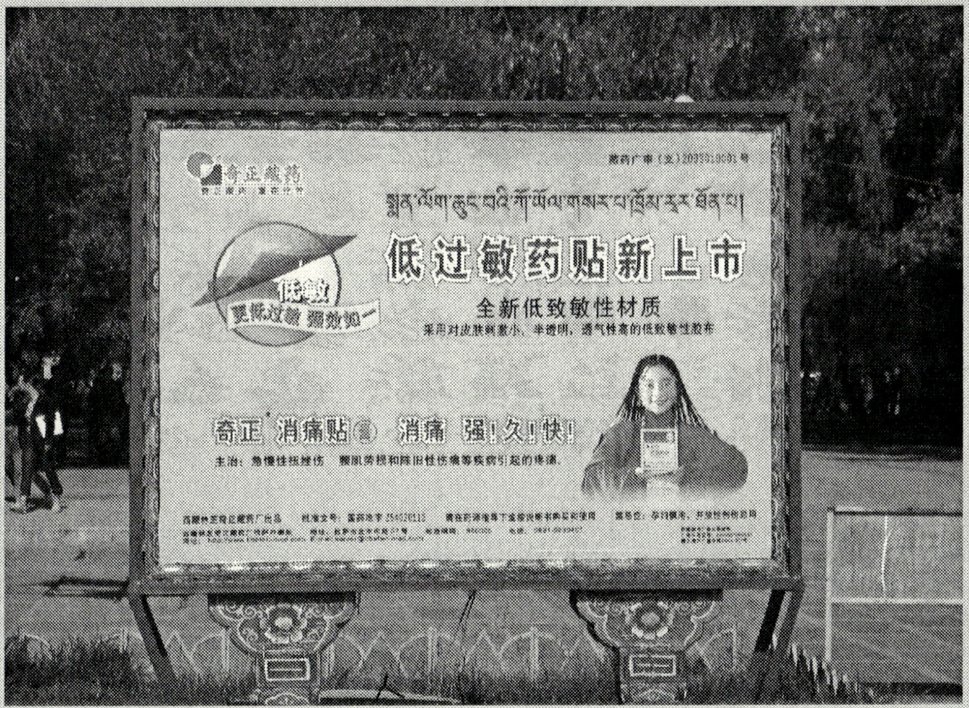

Cheezheng advertisement   ©TIN

The Cheezheng Group states that they produce medicines with speed, utilizing "technology and industrialization." As their website states, "Cheezheng offers the world a brand-new type of traditional Tibetan medicine, making it possible for person to experience the unique effect of Tibetan medicine." Medicinal products produced by Cheezheng are currently being sold throughout the PRC and abroad. Some of their products have been exported to North America, Southeast Asia, and several countries in the European Union. The Group has a staggering 300 million RMB (approx: £19.6million; 28.4million; $36.25million) in assets. In 2001, their annual income from sales was 220 million RMB (approx: £14.4million; 20.8million; $26.6million.) The Cheezheng Group, which includes both Tibetan and Chinese investors, currently owns eight product and procedure patents and has drug registration numbers for 48 kinds of Tibetan medicines. Their products are certified at the ministerial level and recognized by the National Health and Supervision Bureau. At the 26th Geneva International Invention and New Technology Exhibition in April 1998, Cheezheng's Pain Relieving Plaster won the gold invention award, marking the first international honour of its kind given to Tibetan medicine. The Cheezheng Group now operates 25 branches. Visit www.tibetan-med.com for more information on Cheezheng.

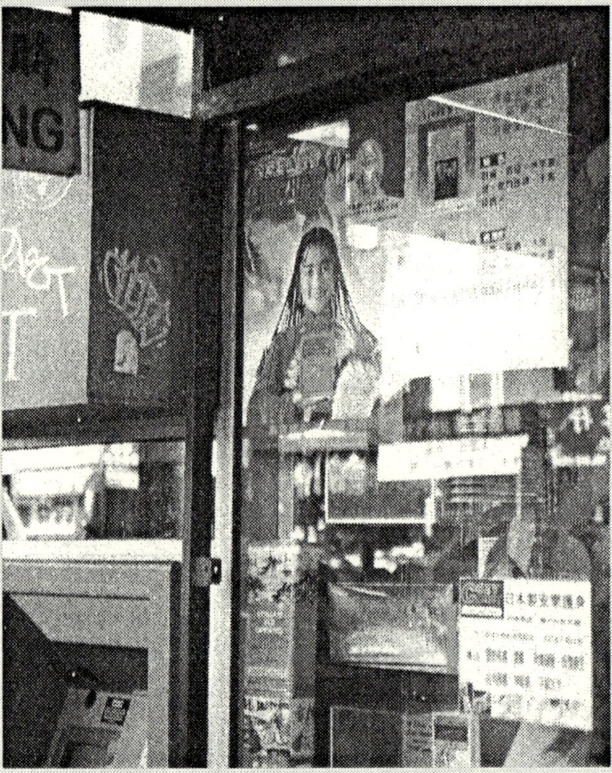

Advertisment for Cheezheng pain relieving plasters in Chinatown, San Francisco, USA   ©TIN

In addition to questions about the quality and harvesting practices of ingredients, production methods themselves have changed substantially. Notions of cleanliness and hygiene in medicine preparation are taking precedent over the quality of plants or other ingredients, harvesting techniques, etc. In some factory settings, particularly among young Tibetan and Chinese executives who are trained in business management rather than *sowa rigpa* practice, there is a palpable embarrassment about 'traditional' methods of production and a greater striving to conform to 'modern' standards. In addition, although ritual *men drup*, or medical empowerments – key elements of traditional Tibetan medical production –

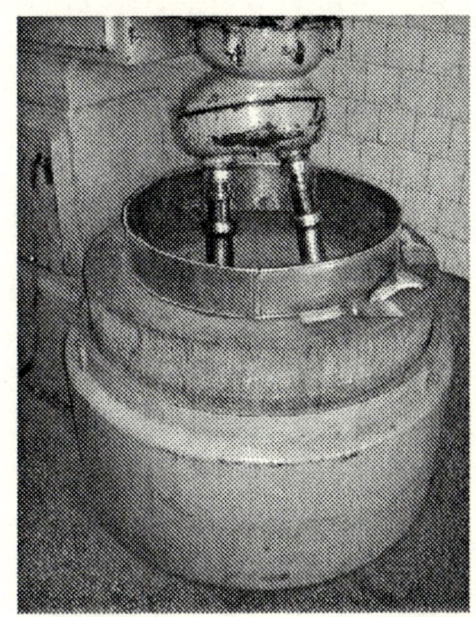

Grinding device   ©TIN

are performed in some state-sponsored and private factories, they have taken a decidedly less important role in the production of medicines. In some factory settings, debates continue about the kinds of machines that should be used to grind herbs and other medicinal ingredients. According to the *Gyushi*, other medical texts and oral tradition, medicinal ingredients should be ground by stone, not by metal, as metals can alter the properties inherent in the ingredients themselves. In some commercial factory contexts, these 'old' stipulations have been disregarded and ingredients are ground by metal blades. In other factories, new grinding machines have been devised in which the machine is powered by electricity and uses metal parts, but the medicine is ground in giant stone mortars and pestles. The processes by which medicinal ingredients are heated (sometimes boiled) and dried have also become similar areas of contention. In some instances, new pressures of standardisation and commercialisation have promoted innovative thinking on the part of Tibetan doctors and others involved in the industry. But the challenges to the future of Tibetan medicine due to the demands of commercial production remain great.

One Tibetan pharmacologist at a large medical factory described the contradictions in production methods and the implications for medical efficacy that surface as a result of the unquestioning implementation of GMP regulations:

> *Take the example of* bu tog, *an earth medicine. The best bu tog comes from the Chang Tang [Tibet's 'northern plains']. Today we get some from China, though the quality is not as good. The problem is that, according to my teacher and our recipes, we should be using aged bu tog that has been put into containers and preserved for a number of years (...) before being used in medicines. But the GMP says that this is not the right way to make medicine, and that all the ingredients need to be fresh. But for us; the older, the better, in this instance. [Using the wrong kind of ingredient, or using it in a way that] does not match our history, the history of making this medicine, creates a problem with efficacy of the medicine itself. This is also the case with preparation of hot and cold medicinal ingredients today.*

According to this Tibetan medical pharmacist and others, working under the new regulations has meant that *amchi* are losing control over their medicines. The GMP as it is applied on Tibetan medicine in the PRC today fundamentally creates a difference in what is meant by 'quality' and 'efficacy.' Yet to most Tibetan doctors – even ones who do not produce their own medicine – the smells, tastes and natures of the ingredients are crucial; this is how quality is determined. The time of collection is also important, as is the state of mind of the collector and the need to consider the amounts that are used. But these considerations are quite different than what GMP means by 'standardization.'[18] As another doctor stated:

> *The GMP doesn't care about these things. They are more concerned with the market situation and living up to the standards set by the government, about making our medicines in airtight rooms, in expensive buildings. According to the GMP, they could collect and use plants even from a place that is at war and it would be okay. You could go to Iraq or Afghanistan and collect things from there and use them in medicines. But to us, this would be very bad, particularly if the people collecting were also engaged in killing and fighting. This would affect the quality of the medicines and benefits of the medicines, too. But they don't think of such things. They think of making sure everything is 'clean' in their way.*

Private, Small-Scale Medicine Production

Private, small-scale production of Tibetan medicine still exists throughout Tibet. However, it may become the exception rather than the rule, like the fate of private clinical practice, as we shall discuss in the next chapter. Changes such as the depletion of natural resources and the GMP standards beacon the certain death of private medical production, and with it the loss of a body of knowledge that integrates ecology, medicine and religious practice, as well as the extinction of 'real' or 'pure' – and therefore most efficacious – Tibetan medicines. Others see the shift from private production to standardised factory production as a step in the direction of true 'modernisation' and the scientific advancement of *sowa rigpa*, toward the aim of sustaining and improving on centuries of medical experience. Others still see the decline of private medicine production as the end to remaining obstacles blocking the complete control of Tibetan medical resources by capitalist interests – even in the name of socialist state medical services and the advancement of one of the PRC's 'national minorities'. Some private practitioners themselves continue to produce medicines that disregard national notions of 'good manufacturing practices' and adhere instead to a different kind of GMP: methods of production passed down orally from their teachers and lineage holders and recorded in old texts, many of which were hidden during the Cultural Revolution, but have since resurfaced.

---

18 For a specific example of such dynamics in the TAR and Switzerland, see Adams (2003) and Schwabl (2003), respectively.

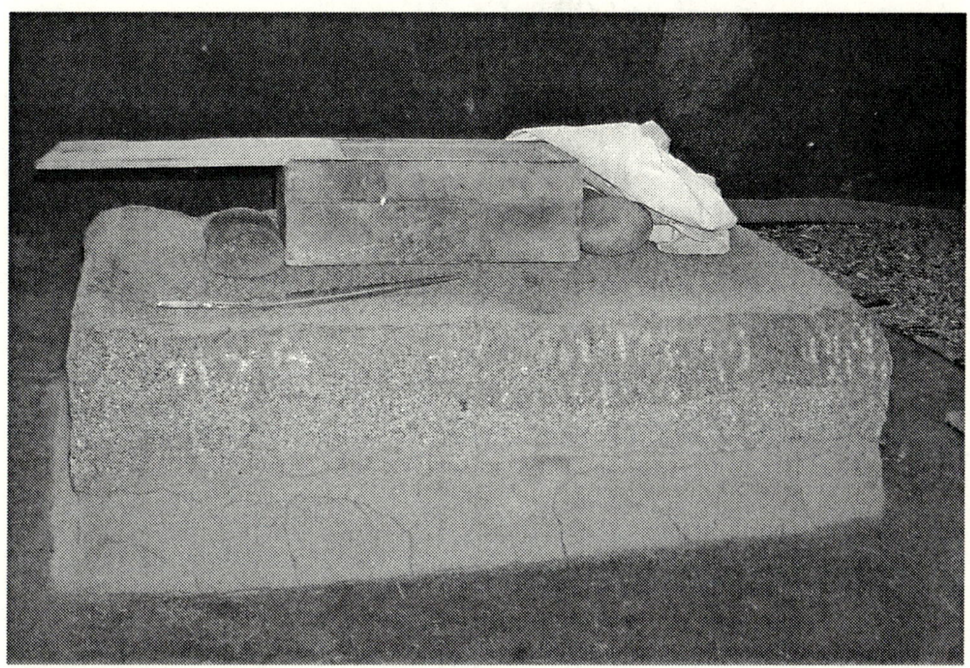

Grinding stone   ©TIN

Regardless, many *amchi* in contemporary Tibet – from private practitioners in remote areas to well-educated scholar-practitioners with secure positions at large urban institutions – speak with a sadness and concern about the separation of those who *produce* medicine from those who *prescribe* medicine in Tibet today. This is the core of what is lost with the decline of private production. The struggles to establish and maintain new standards, as well as to succeed as a for-profit business has meant that fundamental tenets of how Tibetan medicine is supposed to be produced and prescribed are changing. It has also meant that a pharmacopoeia that was once viewed as a means to rebalancing a patient's humours is now beginning to be conceived as a set of drugs, each with drug registration numbers and patents, that are prescribed based on cursory symptoms, or sold over the counter as quite general tonics and remedies. The growing industry of Tibetan medicine is drastically changing Tibetan doctors' relationships to their medicines and their patients – mirroring patterns of medical professionalisation and the rise of pharmaceutical industries in the history of biomedicine and 'western-style' health care. Many Tibetan doctors today also speak of the decreasing knowledge within these larger medical factories about where different medicinal ingredients are coming from, as well as the quality and variations of particular ingredients. This is a ramification not only of the Tibetan medical industry but also of the changes in Tibetan medical education, as we have explored in Chapter Two, and a further lament in regards to the declining numbers of *amchi* who both practice and produce their own medicines.

The commercialisation of Tibetan medicine, particularly the increasing markets for a variety of raw materials, is having an interesting and in some senses paradoxical impact on production and clinical practice at a local level. In some instances, the rise in demand for and price of particular ingredients has made it more difficult for small-scale private practice *amchi* to produce their own medicines. In other instances, *amchi* now have greater access to a wider variety of ingredients than they did in previous generations – that is, if they have the cash to buy them. Road networks both within Tibetan areas of the PRC and between the Tibetan Plateau and the Indian and Nepali Himalayas, for instance, has meant that *amchi* who used to rely on a smaller retinue of *materia medica* can access ingredients that they previously did not use. Today, *amchi* practicing in remote nomadic communities on the Chang Tang might still rely on a small, locally available pharmacopoeia, as well as on external therapies like bloodletting or moxibustion. Their colleagues in the boomtown of Nagchu Prefecture, on the other hand, might have access to a greater range of ingredients than did their fathers or grandfathers. Yet such increased access to ingredients is almost exclusively tied to a cash economy; it also contributes to general inflation of market prices for particular raw materials as well as the continued depletion of rare or endangered species.

Meeting new standards and production demands has also had an impact on the ability of rural practitioners of Tibetan medicine to treat patients, from private practice *amchi* or those who are a part of the government health care system, to those who straddle this divide between private practitioner and public servant. Not only is it becoming more difficult for many private practitioners to produce their own medicines, due to increasing market demand for raw materials and the greater importance of a cash economy, as well as stipulations about standardization of production methods, but it is also becoming more difficult in some regions of the TAR and other Tibetan areas of the PRC for these individual practitioners to buy ready-made Tibetan pharmaceuticals. One township doctor from an agro-pastoral region of central Tibet expressed these dilemmas as follows:

> *We used to make all our medicines. But now, with these big companies and middlemen who pay people to collect plants, we can only make a few kinds of medicines, and it is more expensive to get ingredients. We can't pay people the same prices as those businessmen, and we also want to collect fewer medicines from one place [than they do]. Now we buy medicines from the Mentsikhang factory, but this is a problem because we don't trust the quality. They are more concerned with making profits than with having the right kinds of ingredients. If we give people medicines that don't work well, they think our system of medicine is weak. But that is not true. We have many medicines for many different kinds of illnesses, and ours has fewer side effects than western medicine. We can treat old illnesses better, too. We come from a place that is rich in medicinal plants, but we have less and less chance to actually use these medicinal plants. Aside from this, we do not have the means to buy things like gold or other precious gems for medicines, as well as things like la dzi (musk).*

It is interesting to note that this practitioner is not only a township doctor but also a lineage *amchi*: both his father and his mother had been practitioners of Tibetan medicine. In recent years he had also been given some training in basic biomedical care through an international NGO's training programme. Even though Tibetan medicine could be studied by any member of the masses, he explained, *amchi* who come from a lineage were capable of producing medicines that were more efficacious than those who only had 'school learning.' Likewise, he felt that healers with claim to lineage were more suited to practicing *sowa rigpa*. However, when asked if he had decided to instruct any of his five children in Tibetan medical practice, he replied that they had other ambitions – a comment that points to the connections between changes in Tibetan medical education, Tibetan medicine's place in the overall health care structures in Tibetan areas of the PRC and the notion of a crisis of confidence in Tibetan medical practice.

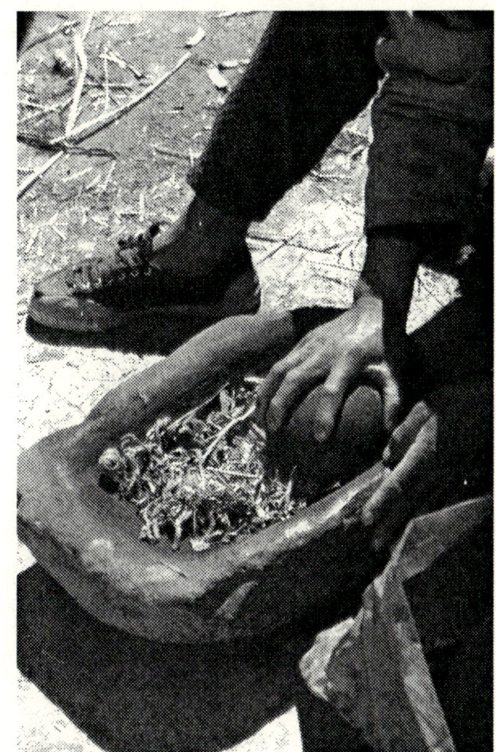

Grinding, traditional style   ©TIN

One Tibetan doctor from northern Nepal described the differences between Nepal and China in terms of access to medical materials, issues of conservation and the impact of the growing international market for ready-made Tibetan medicinals as follows:

> *The big factories in Tibet are taking away the rights of private amchi much more than the conservation organizations and the government here in Nepal. The Nepali government says that amchi don't know what they are doing when they collect and that they and other local people don't know what they are doing by selling all of their raw herbal materials to India. So they have stopped trade in some places, for conservation purposes, and some organizations are trying to teach amchi about conservation or work with them to protect plants from the big businessmen...*

> *But in China-Tibet, the situation is different because it is so much about making a profit from medicines. Private amchi are being pushed out. Only those private amchi who just stay quiet, keeping to themselves and using their small grinding*

> *stones can actually keep making their own medicines. The Chinese want the benefit out of the TAR. Tibetan medicine can make Chinese and Tibetan businessmen even richer. But if they stop private amchi from producing, this just means that there are more medicines to sell to the outside and less to help treat people. Only the ones who make medicines on a very small scale can continue producing medicines, unless they are connected to a factory and have the proper permits. But they are often poor, so they can't buy the ingredients that don't grow in their areas, and therefore also make inferior medicines, not because of any fault of their own knowledge. The Chinese are taking the Tibetan medicine away from Tibetans. They want the benefits of Tibetan culture, but they want to strip Tibetans of their rights and access to amchi and good medicines.*

As much as this *amchi*'s opinion is an apt summary of the state of Tibetan medicine production and its socio-economic effects on the lives of Tibetans, it is worth questioning who the 'they' are in this picture. 'They' certainly are not just the Chinese government or business interests, as many Tibetans are involved in the commercialisation of their medicine. 'They' also should include the consumers of alternative therapies, products that are often ironically described as 'natural' or 'eco-friendly.' Likewise, it would be inaccurate to assume that the only realm of departure from traditional harvesting and production practices is occurring within Tibetan areas of the PRC. On the contrary, the Men-tsee-khang in Dharamsala produces approximately 160 different medications using a hybrid of modern and traditional techniques. They also hire professional collectors to gather medicinal ingredients from places such as Ladakh and Manali. In this context as well, there is a rising set of concerns about the quality and availability of medications because of the rise in factory production, an increasing (global and regional) demand to produce more medicines and decreasing coordination between those who collect ingredients, produce medicine and treat patients.

This shows the importance of carefully adopting and re-interpreting old scriptures and traditions. The need to implement GMP and, at the same time, reacting to the availability of the natural ingredients, present considerable challenges. As we will show in the next chapter, integration with western biomedicine can be added to this list. In particular, the leading institutions of Tibetan medicine have the task of adapting traditional knowledge in a way that safeguards its survival, despite the influx of modern elements. From the governmental side, restrictions on the use of endangered species and on the recognition of Tibetan Medicine as a proper medical system are mandatory. Throughout the geographical range of Tibetan medicine however, different circumstances apply.

In Nepal, restrictions on trade in medicinal plants, national park legislation and policies on use of Non-Timber Forest Products (NTFP), availability of ready-made Tibetan medicines from India and, to a lesser extent, Tibet, as well as the last eight years of political instability and violence have all impacted the regulation of trade and harvesting throughout the Nepali Himalayas. In Mongolia, where there has been a state-sponsored revitalization of *sowa rigpa* since 1990, the main medical factory now produces 200 tons of medicine per year and more than 200 kinds of medicines. Through state and non-governmental support, as well as connections fostered with Tibetan medical communities in India, they have embarked on cultivation and conservation efforts, as well as experiments in medical ingredient substitution. But the Mongolians are also working within inherently limited ecosystems. As with the Tibetan Plateau, Mongolia's high, dry steppe is particularly vulnerable to global environmental change. In this sense, it is worth considering the social and ecological costs of Tibetan medicine in the global marketplace. This is certainly not a black-and-white issue. And Tibetan doctors are often the first to exalt benefits that can come to 'all sentient beings' by increasing global access to *sowa rigpa*. But all of these forces have direct and lasting impact on the very nature of Tibetan medicines within and outside the PRC, and on the ability of future generations of Tibetans to be treated with their medicines, by their doctors.

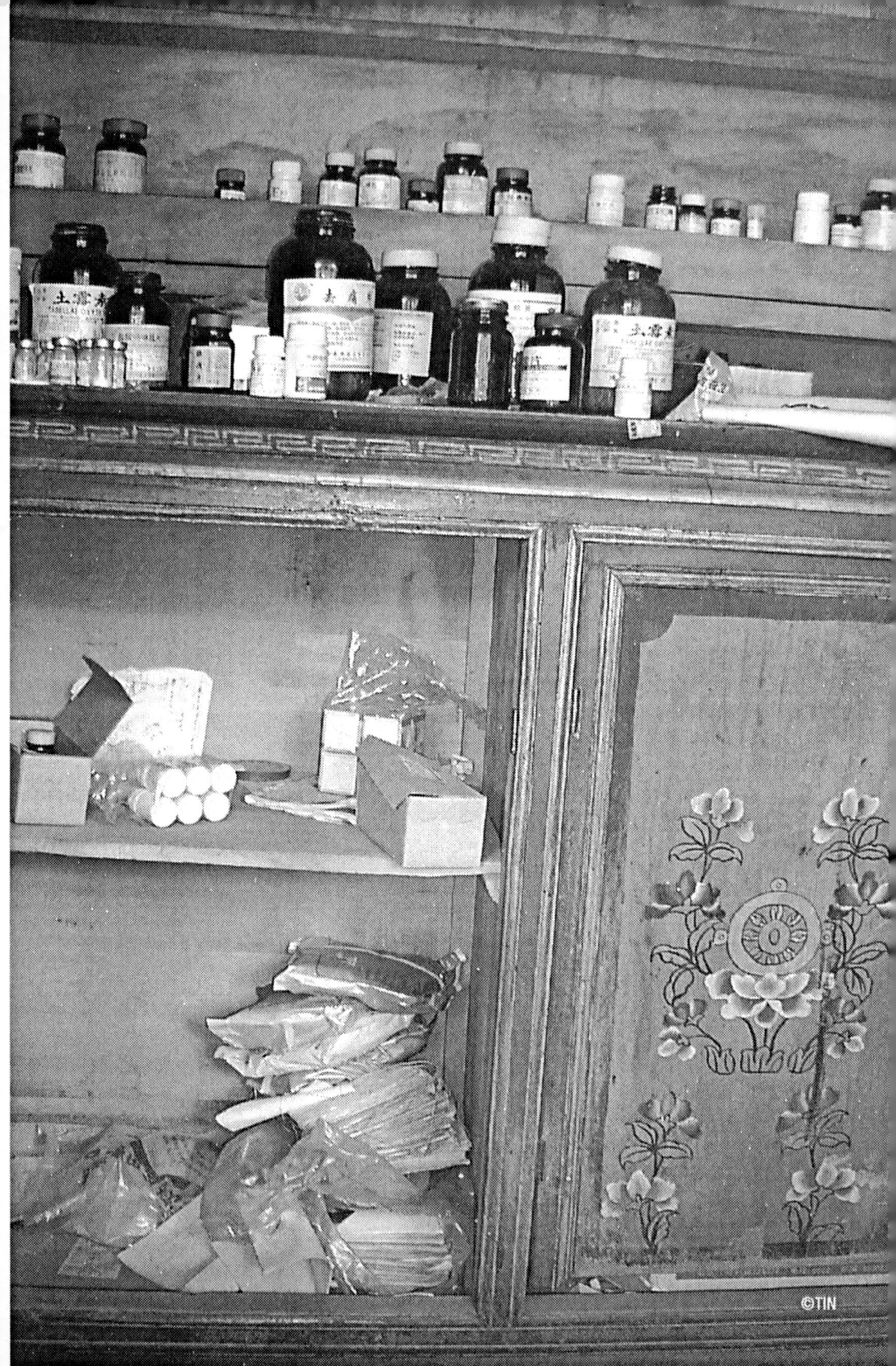

Chapter Four

Clinical Practice: The Crossroads of Tibetan Medicine and Biomedicine

It is noon at the township clinic on a freezing day in April. Snow has been falling steadily since the previous evening and this township – a mixture of Tibetan and Chinese-style buildings along a stretch of muddy, unpaved road – has been blanketed by the snowstorm. But soon the sun will break through cloud cover and the strength of high altitude rays will begin burning through winter toward spring.

The township clinic, one of several larger structures along the road, consists of five rooms made of stone and wood: a clinic and dispensary, a delivery room, an in-patient room, a store room and an office for the three township doctors assigned to this post. The construction, though not entirely traditional, still blends into the hillside abutting this township. Behind the clinic sits a newly built pair of toilets. Cast in tile and cement, the toilets are more typical examples of government construction throughout rural and urban Tibet than the township clinic itself. There is a telephone at this clinic – a novelty for some townships in rural Tibet – and the dispensary is decently, though not plentifully, stocked with both Tibetan and modern pharmaceuticals.

The three township doctors are inside, drinking Tibetan tea and trying to keep warm. One is a woman in her late forties. She explains that she has had very little formal medical training – a one-year course in biomedicine when she was eighteen and no training in Tibetan medicine – but that she has been practicing medicine at this clinic for thirty years. Although she considers herself a general practitioner, the fact that she is the only woman in the hospital has meant that she has assisted more births than her two male colleagues. She has recently received supplemental training in maternal and child health by a foreign NGO's midwife training programme. She is a native of this township, and works with the strength and ease of someone undaunted by the elements and this environment.

The second doctor is a young man originally from western Tibet and a graduate of the Tibetan Medical College in Lhasa. He has been stationed here for two years, and views this assignment as an extension of his medical training. He is more of a 'city boy' than his colleagues, and seems to suffer most from the cold and the lack of facilities. Although he is trained in Tibetan medicine, he has a difficult time practicing out here because the medicines to which he has access are sparse by his standards; Tibetan medicines should be supplied through the county hospital on a regular basis, but he explains that the county hospital itself has a much smaller budget for purchasing Tibetan medications than biomedical drugs. As the most literate of the three doctors, in Chinese and Tibetan, he has found his niche as something of a clinic administrator, placing orders for medicine from the county hospital and helping patients and their families petition for Co-operative Medical System (CMS) subsidies for medical treatment. Some patients come to him expecting to find an adept biomedical practitioner, simply by virtue of his age and his more 'modern' air. But he has admitted his relative ignorance of biomedicine and stuck to his Tibetan medical practice – a fact that has earned him suspicion among the local population, instead of respect.

The third doctor is a middle-aged man dressed in a traditional *chuba*, who the others quickly agree is the most popular of the three clinicians. Like his female colleague, he is from this area, and has had relatively little institutional training in either biomedical or Tibetan medical practice. Yet, he apprenticed with his father, a Tibetan doctor, when he was young, and is adept not only in pulse diagnosis but also makes a few of his own Tibetan medicines, even today. His biomedical training came in the form of a three-year state-sponsored course in the late 1970s; he has since received some additional training from a foreign NGO's health and hygiene outreach program. They say people trust him not only because he is older and comes from a lineage of *amchi*, but also because he has the ability to practice both medical systems. The clinic serves a large, primarily nomadic population to the northeast of Lhasa, much of it off the road; this doctor is comfortable on horseback, and will travel to treat people.

But what of the clinic itself? The delivery room looks nearly abandoned, save an uninviting delivery table and some empty bottles and used syringes in one corner. About ninety percent of local women still choose to give birth at home. The in-patient room is nothing more than a few wooden cots, neat enough, though spare. As in county and prefecture hospitals, family members are expected to bring food and bedding for their sick relatives and to nurse patients themselves. The room used by all three practitioners for diagnosis and treatment is the most tidy of the lot, its rammed earth floor swept clean of mud and snow even at the tail end of a storm. On one wall rests a wooden cabinet painted with Tibetan motifs, in which bottles of *rilbu* and powder medicines are stored. Each bottle and jar is neatly labelled in Tibetan. A number of the containers are empty. An empty cardboard *rinchen rilbu* box has been turned into a dustbin, and a few varieties of these precious pills sit in the cabinet. A metal closet rests against another wall and holds the clinic's biomedical supplies, the most plentiful among them being strong IV antibiotics and glass bottles of glucose, also to be administered intravenously. A dusty poster of Mao, Deng and Zhao is tacked up near the desk that all three doctors share. Most of the space on the desk itself is taken up by stacks of pink CMS receipts, a stethoscope and blood pressure cuff and handwritten record books in which the doctors record births, deaths, and sicknesses – statistics to be collected annually by representatives of the county Health Bureau. Tibetan incense burns in one corner of the room, cutting the smells of bile, dirt and antiseptic.

This description gives one a sense of the terrain of clinical practice in much of Tibet today. Although circumstances vary throughout Tibetan areas of the PRC, most obviously between rural and urban regions, it is rare to find practitioners who deal only in Tibetan remedies, or approach healing solely with the tools of pulse diagnosis, traditional urinalysis, tongue examination and *sowa rigpa*-style patient history. For better or for worse, clinical practice is a hybrid endeavour, and the reality of government support for Tibetan medicine within the state health care structure reveals a complex and sometimes contradictory picture. This chapter is devoted to exploring some of the circumstances under which Tibetan medicine is practiced in both rural and urban clinical settings, in the context of state health care and reform in modern Chinese history. It also addresses some of the reasons why private Tibetan medical practice is declining in both contexts, but also why it persists. Finally, this chapter touches on the rise of clinical research using Tibetan medicines both in the PRC and abroad, and explores the effects that 'proving' Tibetan medical efficacy through biomedical methods and terms is having on this practice in Tibet today.

State Health care and Tibetan Medicine in Rural Communities

The above sketch of life at a township clinic illustrates some of the larger dynamics at work between rural and urban Tibetan communities, and the access to Tibetan medicine in these contexts. Theoretical and clinical innovation within Tibetan medicine is often – though not exclusively – the domain of urban medical practice; yet many people seeking *sowa rigpa* treatment remain rural dwellers who are often unable to travel beyond the county level to seek medical services. For this reason, the circumstances under which Tibetan medicine has been integrated into the state health care system at not only the prefecture but also the county and township level is a crucial piece of our story.

Since 1985, Tibetan medicine has been sanctioned within the health care system of the TAR and from 1993, Tibetan medicine practice had been integrated not only into prefecture-level state-sponsored care, but also at county and sometimes township levels.[19] In 1991, the Mentsikhang reported that health bureaux throughout ethnic Tibetan regions of Chinese provinces, including the TAR, employed more than 1,500 Tibetan medicine doctors.

Although the ratio of population to biomedical physicians in rural Tibet was approximately 1000:1 in the early 1990s, the ratio of population to Tibetan physicians remained almost 5000:1 at the same time – a number that is higher than the national average of population to traditional practitioners.[20] According to a 1999 report on health and health care in Tibet produced by the China Intercontinental Press, by the end of 1995, the TAR boasted 14 Tibetan medicine research institutes and Tibetan medicine departments in more than 60 county hospitals, as well as more than one thousand Tibetan medical providers at that level of care. In addition, the report claims that there

---

19 For instance, by 1993, Lhasa, Shigatse, and Shannan (Lhoka) Prefectures all supported separate Tibetan medical hospitals and medical factories (Janes: 2001: 199-202).

20 Janes (2001: 202), Young (1989), Jamison et al. (1984)

were more than four thousand rural Tibetan medicine doctors working within the health care system.[21] Furthermore, the same report states that 530,000 people visited county and prefecture-level Tibetan medicine hospitals in 1997, comprising 20% of all visits to hospitals in the TAR for that year; the Lhasa Mentsikhang was visited by 198,000 people in that same year.

These statistics paint a relatively hopeful picture of the access rural Tibetans have to Tibetan medical practitioners and treatments. However, the numbers are hard to confirm; it is difficult to know, for instance, if private *amchi* and medico-religious practitioners are accounted for at all in this statistical portrait. A continued demand among rural Tibetans for access to Tibetan medical treatment, as well as the deployment of young practitioners to the countryside after their initial training, suggests that the number of Tibetan medical practitioners in rural settings might continue to grow. Yet, as we have alluded to in Chapter Two and in the introduction to this section, people who are trained solely in Tibetan medicine often face an ambivalent patient population who increasingly associate the power and responsibility of being a doctor with the ability to administer

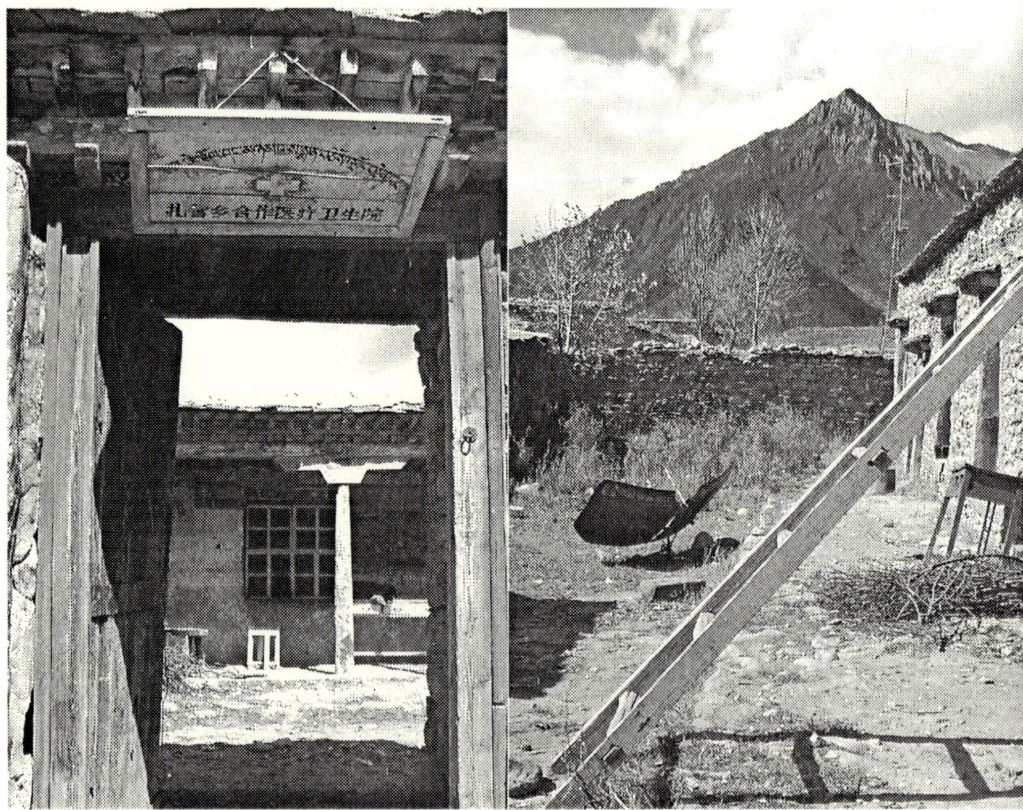

Shang clinic

©TIN

21 Yun (1999: 20)

biomedicines rather than treat with Tibetan medicine and diagnostic methods. Therefore, even though someone might be technically trained as a Tibetan *amchi*, and be counted as such in regional statistics, this does not necessarily mean that he or she practices Tibetan medicine, either partially or exclusively. Indeed, practitioners like the young graduate from the Tibetan Medical College now working at the township clinic described in this chapter's introduction, who refrain from prescribing medicines they have not been trained to use, are rare.

In addition, these statistics do not address the ways that access to Tibetan medicines themselves, at county and township levels, has changed as a result of larger-scale state health care reforms, as well as the impacts that shortages of medicine have had on the ability of people trained in Tibetan medicine to practice in rural contexts. Nor do these statistics account for the history of conflict between urban and rural sectors of the population within China's post-revolution health care systems and between traditional medicine and biomedicine – a national dynamic in which Tibet is also implicated. These dynamics are also tied to economic shifts within the PRC since market reforms began in the 1980s. On the one hand, health policy in the PRC has vacillated significantly between a commitment to universal access and more restricted financing policies. Likewise, the state has, in one respect, celebrated 'traditional' medicines, including *sowa rigpa*, particularly for what they represent in terms of China's cultural richness and its policies on 'national minorities'. And yet, there is also an inherent scepticism or doubt of the medical efficacy of traditional medicines. This scepticism, in turn, facilitates the 'integration' with and domination of biomedicine.[22] On the other hand, market reforms have justified a reduction in funds spent on public health and health care, sometimes forcing hospitals and clinics into market-based activities as a way of generating income to replace lost government funds. In places like Tibet, this has also prompted the decentralisation of control over health bureau budgets from the provincial or prefecture level to county and township levels.

In the TAR, this matrix of tensions has manifested in significant ways: state subsidies of Tibetan medicine continue to decline and health care facilities often engage in profit-oriented business, including the sale of medicine or procurement of special funds from Lhasa or Beijing-based offices interested in 'traditional medicine'; individual patients and a select number of local or regional insurance plans now increasingly cover health care costs, at least for those who can afford to purchase coverage; and in particularly poor rural areas, a patient who has no cash to pay for medical care might not receive any treatment, from Tibetan or biomedical doctors.[23] Indeed, some patients do not even come to township clinics or county hospitals for fear of being turned away due to lack of funds, including lack of an understanding of or access to the Co-operative Medical System. As we shall discuss in more detail below, private practice *amchi* continue to occupy a very important place in community health care – particularly for those patients who either cannot afford to travel to township or county clinics, or who are mistrustful of the CMS state health care system. Such patients will often be treated exclusively by

22 Chen (1989), Janes (2001:203), Adams (2002a)
23 Janes (2001: 205)

private practice lineage *amchi*, if they seek medical care at all. Other patients might seek out health care providers practicing biomedicine, or selling biomedical drugs, in private pharmacies that are on the increase in township or county seats. Some retired state employees now working as private *amchi* support their medical practice – in which payment is not asked for but donations are welcome – by using their government pensions or profit from private trade to buy medicines or raw materials.

Many of the contradictions in access to health care manifest at a local level as confusion over CMS policy. Theoretically, patients who receive both Tibetan and biomedical treatments at township or county facilities are entitled to receive CMS subsidies, in the form of reimbursement, after having paid their annual CMS fee. However, the CMS system itself is relatively new and not well understood or implemented by some counties and townships. Moreover, corruption, budget shortages and social and ethnic dynamics between poor and often illiterate patients and more 'sophisticated' government employees – sometimes including a bias against Tibetan medicine as a 'backwards' form of healing tied to 'superstitious' folk beliefs – further impacts access to clinical Tibetan medicine for rural people through the state health care system. In some contexts, Tibetan medicine is becoming harder to get and more expensive when prescribed. These circumstances depend not only on the predilections and clinical experience of local health care providers – and the interactions between state health care providers and private practice *amchi* – but also on the degree to which local realities and CMS policies converge. This, combined with declining expertise in and resources for locally produced Tibetan medicines, as well increasing government control over the production methods and prices of medicines themselves, has meant that access to quality clinical *sowa rigpa* treatment in rural Tibetan communities is decreasing in some areas. As one township-level *amchi* described:

> *With western medicines, the government supplies our clinic. We order what we need from the county every month. But for Tibetan medicine, we have to supply it ourselves or ask the county doctors to buy it for us. There is often no budget for this, and so it makes it harder for us to treat people with Tibetan medicine. They say Tibetan medicine costs should be covered by the CMS. But often it is not. It is best for our patients if we can use Tibetan medicine and western medicine together, depending on the sickness, and especially for old people and patients with chronic illnesses. But this is becoming less possible.*

In other contexts, the opposite is true. Some academic and popular accounts about the interface between traditional medicine and biomedicine argue that use of 'traditional' remedies increases when government subsidies for health care decrease, partially because traditional medicines are cheaper and more readily available from private sources. In the case of Tibet, particularly in cities, some health professionals, scholars and local people have suggested this trend as well: more people are seeking out Tibetan medicines because they are either cheaper, are more readily available or require less interaction with state health care authorities than access to biomedicine. At this point, it

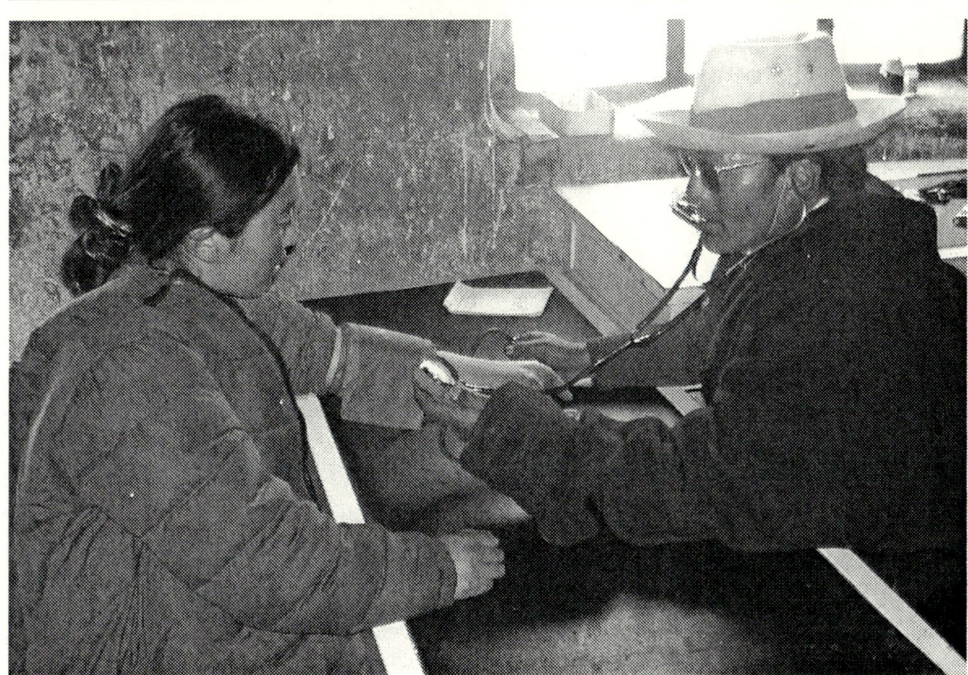

Measuring blood pressure ©TIN

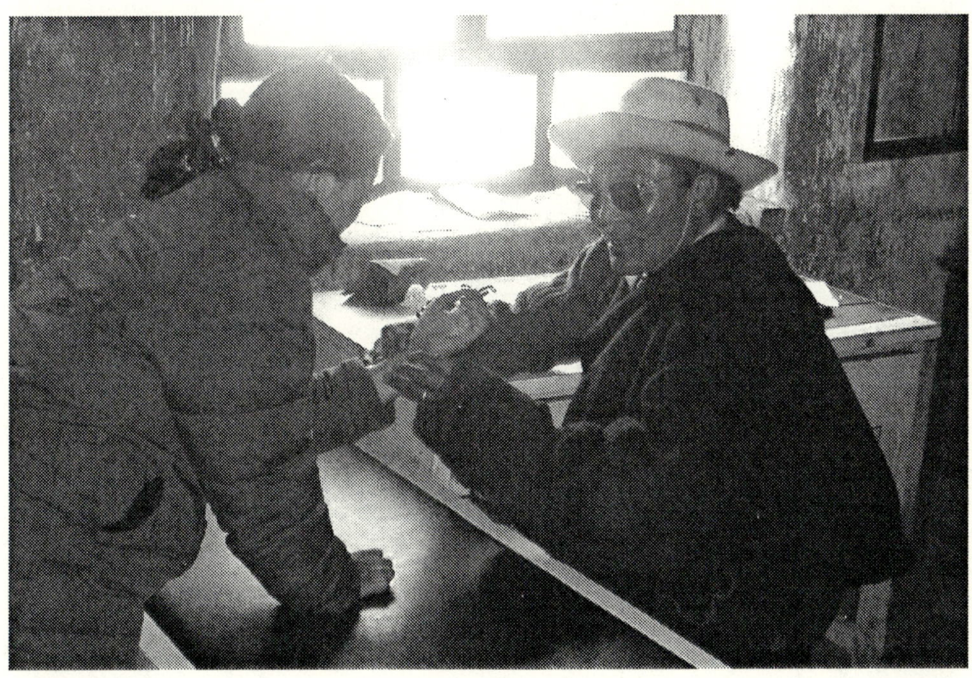

Taking pulse ©TIN

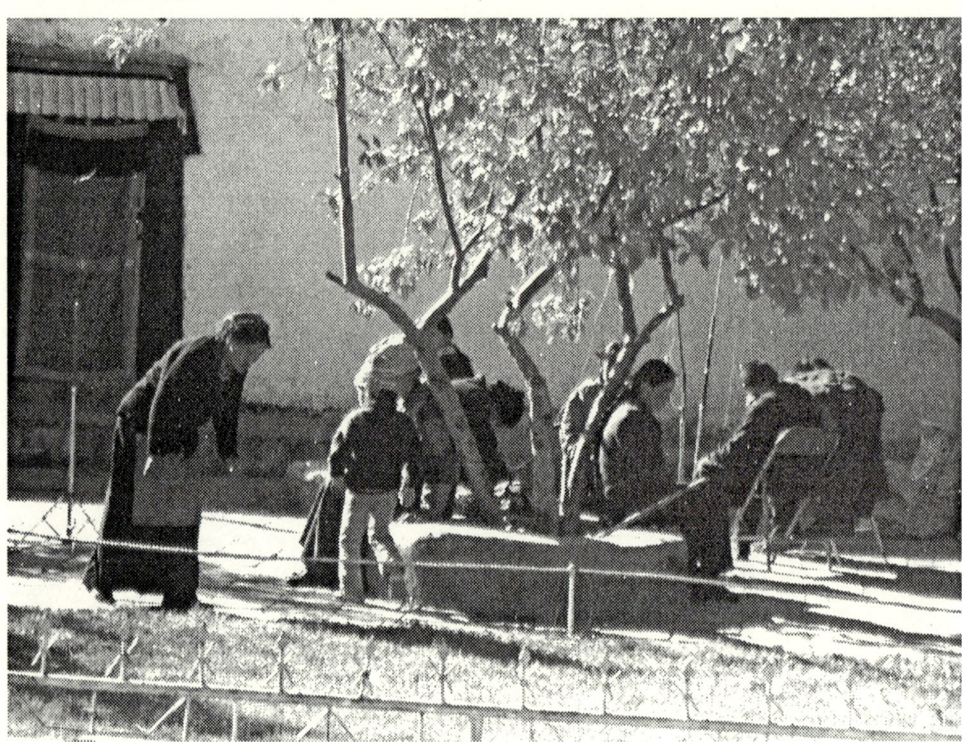

Patients receiving IV drips at Tashi Lhunpo Clinic, Shigatse   ©TIN

is difficult to assume that one view is *the* correct assessment. However, it will be important to monitor price fluctuations in both Tibetan and western medicines over the coming years, to watch the developing relationship between the biomedical juggernaut of big pharmaceutical companies and the Tibetan medical industry, and to see how or to what extent this is impacting Tibetans' choices of and access to health care.

Above and beyond these issues is the interaction between doctors and patients themselves: an encounter often loaded with history, hopes, and fears regardless of the medical system being used. Throughout rural Tibet, it is rare to find a medical practitioner, whether Tibetan or biomedical, who thoroughly examines a patient (physical contact beyond pulse diagnosis or taking someone's blood pressure is rare) or who asks questions of other doctors when they are unsure of the cause or treatment of an illness. For reasons ranging from shyness, inexperience, pride, a lack of biomedical diagnostic technologies or insecurity about their ability to correctly diagnose by Tibetan pulse or urine analysis, some providers leap from hearing a patient describe symptoms to prescribing medicines with little time or energy devoted to diagnosis, from either a biomedical or a Tibetan medical perspective. Although this leap from symptoms to a regimen of drugs can appear to 'work' in the context of biomedicine, partially because of the sheer potency of biomedicines, skipping diagnostic procedures within Tibetan medicine can result not only in misdiagnosis but also in the persistence of an illness.

According to some practitioners of Tibetan medicine, this can, in turn, foster within the general population a sense that Tibetan medicine is not as beneficial or powerful as biomedicine.

When asked about their preferences for medical treatment, many Tibetans will say that they do seek out Tibetan medical care, but not exclusively. Some say that injections are more powerful than pills and that biomedicine is good because it works quickly, while others say that Tibetan medicine is more beneficial because it addresses the root cause of disease, and that it does so without the side-effects of biomedicine. In rural areas, villagers often express the appeal of biomedicine in dramatic terms: it is a system that works well in emergencies and that can produce miracle results, but that can often be 'poisonous,' causing as much harm as good if administered incorrectly. Others say that they would seek out Tibetan medical treatment more if it were regularly reimbursed by CMS, if they knew that medicines were locally made and they could trust the efficacy and potency, or if 'expert' urban Tibetan doctors came to their area and provided clinical treatment that they could trust. Indeed, this latter model of Tibetan medical care is something that has been facilitated by a few foreign NGOs working in Tibet, and has helped, in some instances, to both restore local confidence in the use of Tibetan medicine and also provide opportunities for graduates of prestigious institutes of Tibetan medicine to gain more clinical experience.

In addition to these forces, we must not lose sight of the overall impacts that the commodification of Tibetan medicine and the creation of large factories have also had on the ability of rural Tibetans to receive Tibetan medical care.

From Pulse Diagnosis to Ultrasounds: Urban Clinical Care[24]

A typical Monday morning at the out-patient Mentsikhang in Lhasa, just off the Barkhor, reveals a bustling scene. Patients crowd the downstairs waiting rooms, file through the halls of the Women's Division or seek out doctors specialising in kidney or liver imbalances. Some are urban dwellers, while others are just in from the countryside. On the streets outside the facility one is more likely to see several Chinese people for each Tibetan; inside the Mentsikhang the demographics reverse themselves. Outside, the sound of Chinese language dominates; inside Tibetan is heard more frequently and with great variation: an eastern Tibetan dialect here, a nomad speaking in his northern Tibetan tongue there. On the ground floor, Tibetan medical pharmacists dispense *rilbu* and powders from wooden drawers, folding them into neat packets of paper on which they write or draw (for non-literate patients) the timing and dosage. Across the foyer sits the biomedical dispensary, which is organised in a similar manner, though medications come in plastic packages and metal tubes containing capsules, pills and ointments. Upstairs, doctors and nurses bustle through the halls, traditional Tibetan dresses, *chuba*, swishing

---

24 The information contained in this section in particular draws from the work of Adams and Li (forthcoming 2004).

under white lab coats, stethoscopes as necklaces. Visits with doctors are usually a quick affair, even with some of the elder and most skilled *amchi*. Though each patient will have his or her pulses read by the attending doctor. and sometimes by a novice, full diagnoses often include lab tests and the use of other biomedical technologies. Other times, patients are referred to the in-patient facilities or another Lhasa hospital for further diagnosis or treatment.

When asked, some patients at the Mentsikhang say they seek out care at this facility because they trust in Tibetan medicine more than biomedicine, have an 'old' illness that they feel will be more effectively treated with Tibetan medicine or are suffering from an imbalance that cannot be addressed, or even understood, in biomedical terms.[25] Others don't have much of a preference for the kind of medicine they are given – indeed most are too shy to ask questions about their courses of treatment – but come to the

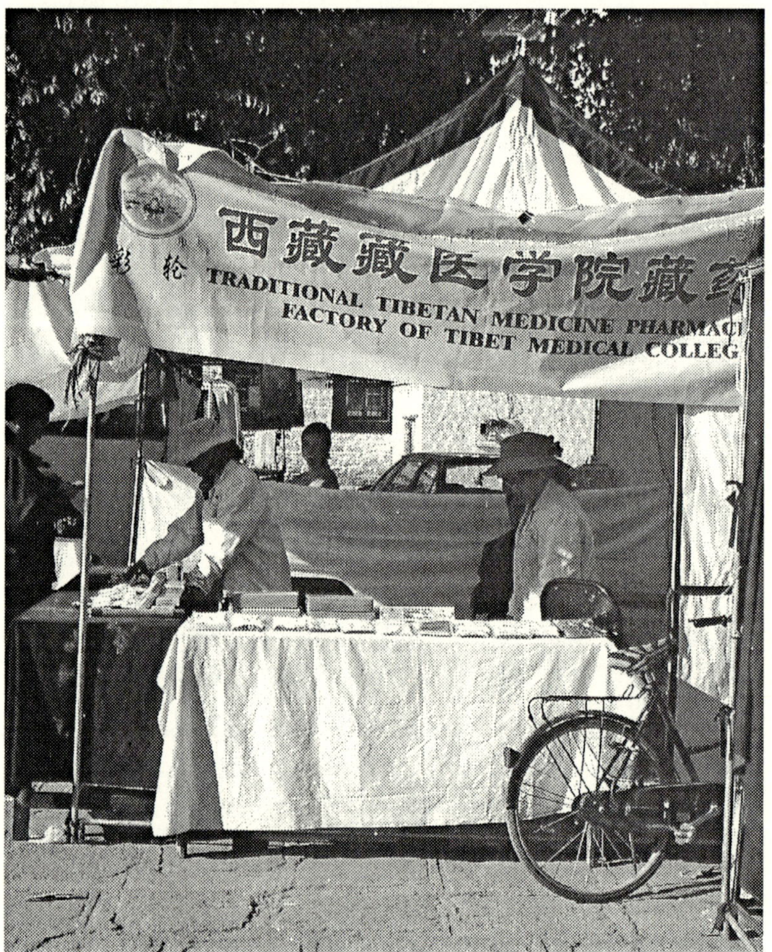

Sale of medicine in front of the Potala ©TIN

25 Several scholars of Tibetan medicine have written about the issue of translation – or untranslatability – between Tibetan medical and biomedical symptoms and illness causality. For more information on this topic, see the work of Adams and Li, Janes, Gerke, Husted and Rapgay, and Jacobson listed in the bibliography.

Mentsikhang because they believe the doctors are more compassionate and approachable than providers at the biomedical facilities in Lhasa. Some patients seek out care at the Mentsikhang because they speak no Chinese and are worried about encountering doctors at other Lhasa hospitals who will not or cannot speak with them solely in Tibetan. Indeed, the language of biomedicine in Tibetan areas of the PRC is Mandarin Chinese: it is the language of government policy, names for medications, as well as the lens through which biomedical concepts of pathology, epidemiology and even physiology, are articulated – even though all hospitals include Tibetan-speaking staff. For non-bilingual Tibetans, this means that the vocabulary of biomedicine, from public health to personal hygiene, remains difficult to decipher. That being said, government agencies and NGOs have begun to produce more health publications that are written in Tibetan as well as Chinese, particularly for use in rural health outreach programmes.[26] Yet, in many respects, doctors at the in-patient and out-patient Mentsikhang facilities, and at many prefecture-level hospitals of Tibetan medicine in other parts of Tibet, function not only as health care practitioners working between medical systems, but also as interpreters of the language of healing for their patients: crossing the lines between *loong* imbalances and tuberculosis tests, between spirit attacks and postpartum haemorrhage, in their efforts to make illnesses surmountable and wellness comprehensible. Particularly at out-patient facilities, many urban Tibetan doctors also function as health educators in a more mundane sense: offering advice and explanations about such things as birth control, sexually transmitted infections and dietary habits. Yet the language that out-patient Mentsikhang doctors speak to each other, particularly those doctors who are in their early forties or younger, is a language that is often structured by biomedical and western scientific concepts. And their practice relies heavily on biomedical technologies. This shift is even more apparent at the in-patient Mentsikhang, where some providers have no formal training in *sowa rigpa* and where doctors have come to rely on ultrasound machines, the laboratory, and routine biomedical examination methods. While *amchi* in rural areas often rely on Tibetan medical diagnostic techniques even if they treat with a combination of biomedicines, the reverse is often the case in urban settings like the Mentsikhang. Lab tests and other biomedical technologies are relied upon in these settings, in part because they are perceived to be more 'accurate' or even 'easier' to use – or to master – than more traditional pulse diagnosis or urinalysis. In the best case scenarios of 'integrated' medicine, biomedical forms of diagnosis do not erase or invalidate Tibetan medical forms, but can reinforce a primary diagnosis done in the manner of *sowa rigpa* practice. However, sometimes these two forms of diagnosis can come into conflict, contributing to a crisis of confidence in Tibetan medicine by both practitioners and patients.

The role of both language and technology is particularly striking when considering how diseases are named and symptoms interpreted in this realm of 'integrated' medicine at institutions like the Mentsikhang. Sometimes the relationship between Tibetan and

26 In addition to government publications, the KunDe Foundation and the Canadian International Development Agency (CIDA), both based in Lhoka Prefecture, TAR, and the Swiss Red Cross (Shigatse Prefecture, TAR), have produced a number of Tibetan-language illustrated texts and posters for use in rural and urban health outreach. The Burnet Institute's HIV/AIDS prevention outreach programmes in the TAR have also produced such materials. OneHEART has produced a bi-lingual Tibetan-Chinese manual for midwife training of township doctors. The Bridge Fund has subsidized the translation and publication of *Where There is No Doctor* into Tibetan.

biomedicine means the creation of one-to-one correspondences between named Tibetan medical conditions and biomedical diseases. This does not necessarily mean that practitioners of each medical system share a conception of simple diseases, but rather that, as two scholars have put it: *"linguistic translation could be deployed as a placeholder for assumptions about a shared perception of symptoms. Correspondences can emerge from deciphering a 'match' of the most obvious forms of symptoms related to differently named diseases described by a patient. Likewise, if symptoms can be eradicated by using either Tibetan or biomedicines, then this shared assumption about diseases and the translatability of illnesses across medical systems can be, in a sense, confirmed."*[27] Things get tricky, however, when either Tibetan trained or biomedically trained physicians at the Mentsikhang perceive the other's diagnosis to be partial at best or even 'wrong'. Although outright confrontations between Mentsikhang doctors on such issues tend to be avoided, particularly in front of patients, the assumptions inherent in drawing parallels between ideas of pathology and treatment in Tibetan and biomedicine can cause problems in clinical practice. Furthermore, the more practical and theoretical experience practitioners have in both systems of medicine, the harder it can become to truly 'integrate' two modes of practices. Likewise, in such 'integrated' settings it is rare to find instances in which biomedical practitioners assume or accept that they have something to learn from Tibetan medicine. Rather, Tibetan medicine is often assumed to be less sophisticated or more rudimentary – and Tibetan medicines slower to work – than biomedicine.

Yet the circumstances of such 'integrated' practice should not simply be perceived as entirely negative, or always interpreted as an affront on the integrity of Tibetan medicine as a system. One of the main benefits of this hybrid approach has been a growing commitment to the Women's Division of the hospitals, including the ability of doctors at the Mentsikhang to perform caesarean sections and handle other difficult deliveries, but to do so within a cultural and linguistic context that feels

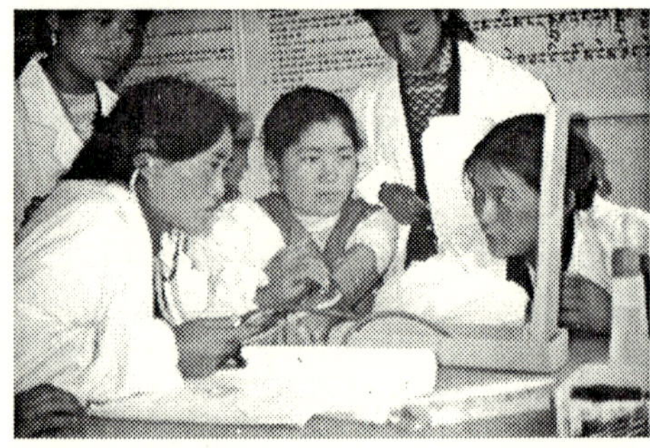

Rokpa clinic in Kham   ©TIN

more 'safe' and trustworthy to many Tibetan women, particularly those from rural areas. Generally speaking, Tibetan patients tend to trust the bedside manners of health care practitioners at the Mentsikhang, or other Tibetan medical hospitals, more than those at the strictly biomedical establishments. There is an assumption (not always validated in practice) that health care providers at Tibetan medical hospitals or clinics will be more compassionate than their equivalents at biomedical hospitals. Some patients connect this better bedside manner with the benefits of Tibetan medicine as a system: that it takes into account, indeed connects, a person's mental and spiritual well-being in

---

27 Adams and Li (forthcoming 2004: 14)

relation to physical wellness. Here, we can hear echoes of complaints often voiced in western countries about the ways biomedical practices can separate a disease from the person it inhabits, or the heart-mind from the body of a patient. Rural patients in particular associate places such as the Mentsikhang with a tolerance for their cultural beliefs and practices; seeking care at such institutions limits their fears about being reprimanded for 'backward' beliefs or behaviours.

In order to illustrate some of these dynamics both between Tibetan doctors and their patients and between *sowa rigpa* and biomedicine in urban clinical contexts, let us take an example from the Women's Division of the outpatient Mentsikhang. This is a particularly apt example, since Tibetan medicine historically did not include many procedures or treatments for women's illnesses, and the increasing numbers of female *amchi* is a relatively modern phenomenon.

Today the Women's Division is crowded. A female Tibetan doctor in her early fifties is the head clinician on call this afternoon. She has not received any formal biomedical training, though she has become familiar through practice with a number of biomedical drugs, which she prescribes on a regular basis. In addition, she has come to rely on lab work when diagnosing a majority of her patients, though she spends more time taking pulses – and takes them with more confidence – than her younger colleagues. In a lull between patients, she explains that medical efficacy comes not only from diagnosing humoral imbalance and prescribing accordingly, but also through the doctor/patient dynamic itself. She speaks about how different this is from: *looking for a disease, naming it and then treating on that basis without considering the specifics of the person, like western doctors.* Yet she admits that she has become comfortable practicing in this way as well. She also says that the type of medicine she prescribes often depends on the patient:

> *Sometimes there are patients who want an instant solution, whether it is from an upset stomach or healing a tear in the women's organs that happened during delivery. They are the kind of patients who only want injections. We don't see many patients like this because they will mostly seek out the biomedical hospitals, but we do see some. Then there are the patients who come here because we know Tibetan medicine, which they trust, or because many of our younger doctors are trained in both kinds of medicine. I am only trained as a Tibetan doctor, but I do know a bit about western medicine as well. When I have questions, I can ask those doctors trained in western medicine who work at the in-patient facility.*

The next patient who enters the room is a woman who has had difficulty conceiving, and who lost her first husband as a result. She has been trying different kinds of therapies (Tibetan, Chinese and biomedical) but she is worried that she won't be able to get pregnant. The doctor spends more time talking with her than examining her, but does perform a basic pelvic exam behind a curtain. She says at the end of the exam that the woman needs to make sure that her sem (heart-mind) is kept peaceful and happy, and

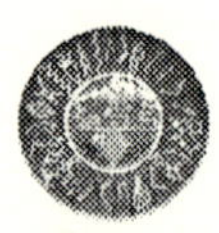

西藏自治区藏医院是国家中医药管理局批准的全国示范藏医医院，也是西藏自治区集医疗、科研、教学、藏药生产为一体的综合性藏医医院。2000年获全国卫生系统先进集体称号。

医院分设门诊部、住院部、藏药厂和藏医药研究所，设300张床位，年门诊量达20多万人次。

根据藏医特点，设有心脑血管病专科、胃肠病专科、肝病专科等10个临床科室。医院现有国家级专家1名、自治区级专家4名，正副主任医师25名，全院职工500多人，形成了一支强大的藏医药科技队伍。

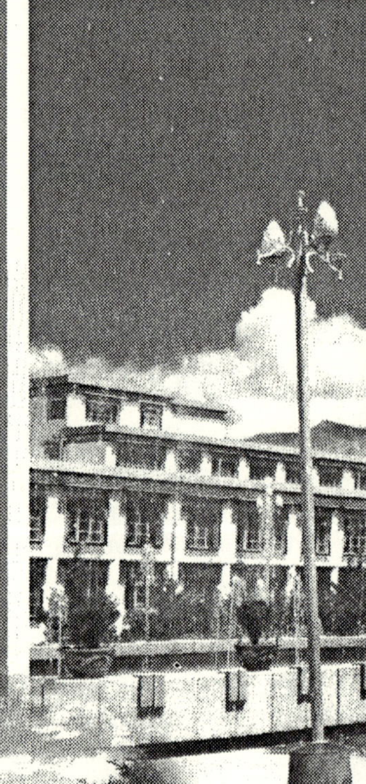

From an advertising brochure for the new Tibetan Medical Hospital, Lhasa

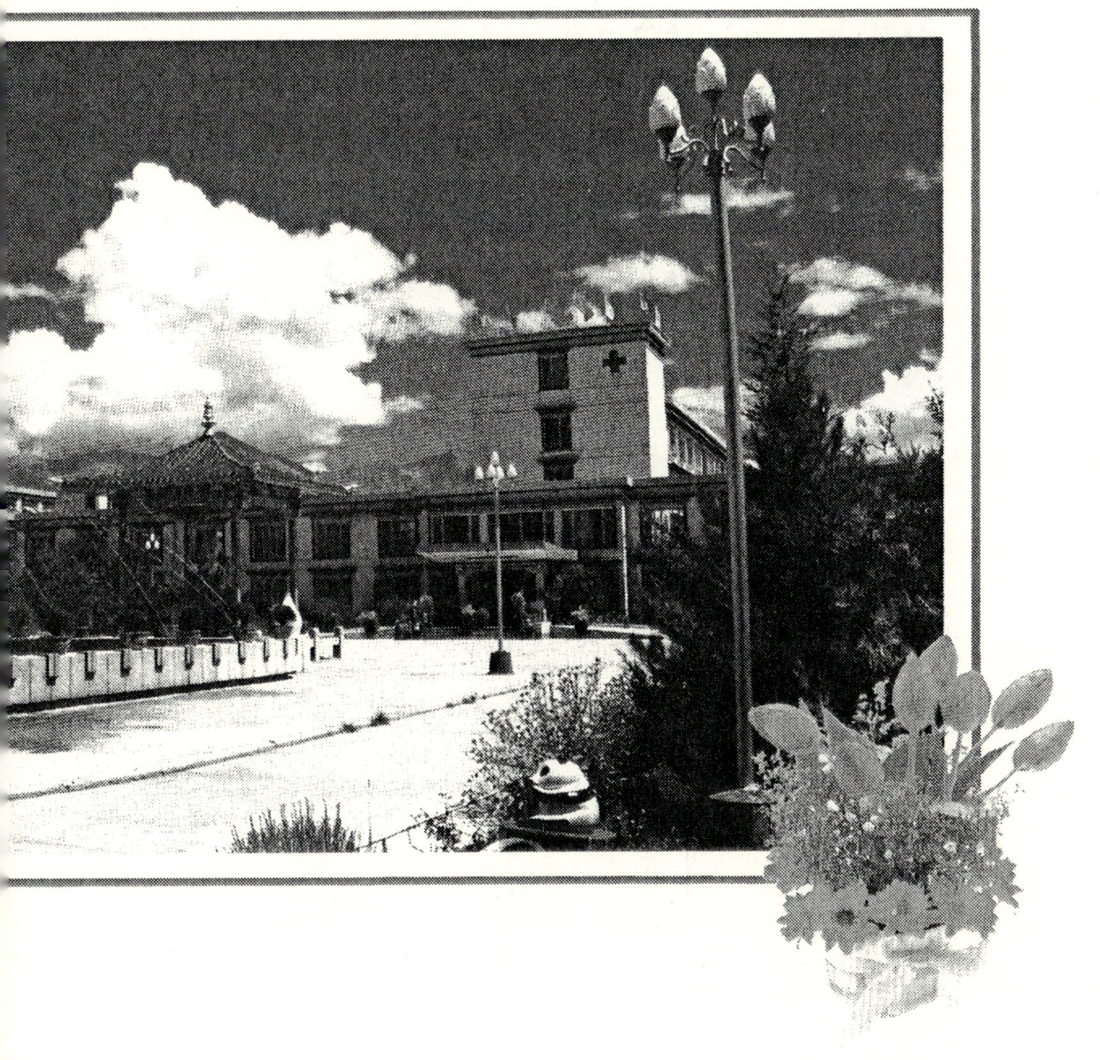

stresses the connection between sem and sugpo, heart-mind and body: *Staying happy and making sure you keep a positive attitude...are very important. The two are related. I can do some things to help increase the chances that you will conceive, but if you have no hope that you will, then you won't.* As she talks, the doctor also prescribes a few different Tibetan medicines for the female patient. They talk a bit more about the woman's working and living conditions. It turns out that her work unit is a road construction crew; she spends many months labouring in climates that are harsh. The doctor confirms the patient's sense that the hard work in difficult environments is reducing her fertility, and she urges her to rest and consider finding another job, if possible.

As the hospital prepares to close for the day, this Mentsikhang *amchi* reiterates the importance of the relationship between doctor and patient, as well as between mind and body, in the healing process. She says that she spends a lot of her time simply counselling young women or couples about different aspects of sex, STDs, contraception, etc, as well as about issues such as diet and behaviour in relation to health. She concluded by saying: *After twenty-five years of women's health experience, I am convinced that to have a clear and good mind and to talk honestly with my patients about what I know is a large part of my responsibility as a doctor. Sometimes that is more important than what medicine I choose to give. Besides, communication can also be medicine.*

The Place of Private Practice[28]

Given the pressures and changes occurring in the realm of public health care, it is perhaps not surprising to learn that private practice Tibetan doctors are becoming more difficult to encounter in some parts of Tibet, or, even if they are present in a given community, are having a more difficult time surviving economically. Many of the issues discussed in Chapter Two, in relation to private instruction in *sowa rigpa*, also hold true for clinical practice in private settings. Indeed, the marriage of theoretical and practical knowledge of Tibetan medicine is a hallmark of the master-apprentice type of relationship. That being said, private practitioners do exist throughout Tibet, in a variety of settings. As discussed in Chapter Two, some are medico-religious practitioners who specialise in specific kinds of medicine, and who are quietly sought out not only by disciples but also by patients, in urban and rural settings. Others are people who might be from a lineage of *amchi* but who have also received advanced institutional training and who set up private clinics. Such clinics are more often encountered in urban areas than rural environments, primarily because the bustle of a city and the diversity of urban populations demand, support, and shelter a diversity of medical practices.[29] In addition, medical clinics built within monasteries provide hybrid private-public and Tibetan-biomedical health care.[30] These clinics are public in the sense that monasteries in

---

28 Published works, conversations with individuals in Tibet, and communications with scholars of Tibetan medicine inform this section. In particular, we would like to acknowledge the ongoing research and observations of a number of scholars, some of whose work is listed in the bibliography and some of whose names remain anonymous in this publication.
29 The Nyarongchen family clinic in Lhasa is an example of a private clinic with a long history and vibrant present-day practice.
30 The clinic at Tashi Lhunpo monastery in Shigatse is an example of such an institution.

contemporary Tibet are usually state-run institutions whose monks and nuns are officially government employees; yet they often operate very differently from county or township clinics and sometimes receive supplemental private funding or medical supplies, sometimes through foreign NGOs, other times through individual sponsors. They also might include a small factory of Tibetan medicine, with proceeds from the sale of medicine helping to fund the clinic itself. At this time, it is unclear what will happen to these factories in coming years, in relation to both GMP standards and the issues surrounding drug registration. Regardless of the actual level and kinds of medical education monk-doctors (or nuns) have received, or the quality of care available at these institutions, monastery clinics are often sought out by the lay population, perhaps because of an inherent trust in the monastery as an institution, perhaps because such choices allow them to express an aspect of their social and religious identity, even if the health care they actually receive in the clinic is limited to being hooked up to an IV drip.

Although there are still *sowa rigpa* practitioners who practice privately in both rural and urban areas, in some senses *amchi* in the countryside can be seen as more susceptible to government scrutiny than their urban counterparts. Both biomedical and Tibetan medical providers at the village and township level must report directly to the county hospital and health bureau director. This creates a level of state control over the practice of Tibetan medicine that does not exist in the same way in more urban environments. These circumstances also make it more difficult for private practice *amchi* to survive. There are several reasons for this. First, this structure increases the explicit ties between state health care policy and Tibetan medical practice, and ties Tibetan medicine to biomedical models of monitoring, standards and control. This reality has both social and economic implications. It is becoming more difficult for private Tibetan medical practitioners to make a living, not only because of the shifting economics of medicine production and raw materials trade, but also because of the predominance of state health care, for better or for worse. Second, it is rare to find a county health bureau or hospital director who is trained in Tibetan medicine, though many are ethnically Tibetan. As such, Tibetan medicine is often only given a confined space, literally and figuratively, in which to be practiced. Tibetan medicines are prescribed for those health ailments for which *sowa rigpa* is perceived as being most effective, such as gastrointestinal disorders, arthritis-like conditions, high blood pressure and mental disorders. Tibetan medical practice can exist within the county hospital or township clinical setting, but the perceived legitimacy of and the mandate for a health care provider to practice *only sowa rigpa*, and to practice in private settings, can be viewed as medically and politically suspect, depending on context. In other words, the fact that someone would *choose* to be treated by a private *amchi* who is perhaps also a renowned religious practitioner, could incriminate both patient and healer, depending on their political reputation and personal history. Of course, there are counter-examples to this trend, often facilitated by the sheer remoteness of some of Tibet's inhabited spaces. Sometimes private-practice *amchi* continue to collect ingredients, make medicines, see patients and teach students without much state intervention at all, simply because they exist at the political and geographic margins or because they have good local political connections.

In this discussion of clinical practice in both rural and urban settings, and in relation to private and public servants, it is worth considering the ways that PRC government health policy and the recommendations and practices of many foreign NGOs begin to mirror each other – even though there is often a great difference in the kinds of medical practices that these parties advocate and the steps they see as necessary to improve health in Tibet. The strengths and weaknesses of both biomedicine and Tibetan medicine are acknowledged: biomedicine is advocated for emergency treatment and epidemic prevention, while Tibetan medicine is seen as appropriate treatment for chronic imbalances. State as well as NGO interventions are sometimes designed on this premise, and there are many ways this combination of therapies can have practical, beneficial results. Just like the 'integrated' curricula we discussed in Chapter Two, this integration of Tibetan and biomedical practice in rural settings is seen as the most positive solution to supporting Tibetan culture as well as increasing quality of life and reducing mortality and morbidity among Tibetan populations. However, the social, political and economic force of biomedicine – the power imbedded in the idea of what it means to save a life in an emergency situation as well as the beneficial aspects of public health regimes – has been a crucial factor in the crisis of confidence in Tibetan medicine and has also contributed to the decline of private Tibetan medical practice.

Another reason for the decline in private practice links social and economic changes. Historically, it was rare to find an *amchi* who would directly charge patients or set fees for their services. An *amchi* might set a sliding scale of prices for medicines themselves, which could be paid for in cash or in kind, but patients paid *amchi* for their services at their discretion and *amchi* functioned more on the premise that their medical practice was a vocation or a religious and spiritual duty, rather than a profession. Although socio-economic divides between different strata of pre-1959 Tibetan society impacted on peoples' access to physicians, and although the Mentsikhang, for instance, has increasingly grown concerned with public health measures, the divide between private and public health care was conceived of differently in historical Tibet.[31] Today, the structure of state health care, changing expectations among patients about what medicine is or what healing means, access to medicinal ingredients or medicines themselves and shifting economies away from barter and toward cash converge to further limit the ability of many private practitioners to survive.

And yet, private practice does continue, in a variety of forms and locations; some even say there are more such practitioners now in certain Tibetan areas than there were twenty years ago. Among nomadic communities in the Chang Tang, in the administrative centres of places like Nagchu and Ngari Prefectures, as well as in private homes from Lhasa to Xining, *amchi* continue to treat patients and make medicines, often *but not always* combining attention to physical and spiritual well being of their patients and adhering closely to the guidelines set by the *Gyushi* or *Bumshi* for the 'Healer Physician'. Many do not drink alcohol or eat meat, for instance, and a sense of private religious

31 Beckwith (1979) discusses this issue of remuneration for health care services in historical Tibet, as well as the denial of health care to poor or lower-caste Tibetans, including Tibetan Muslims. This issue of payment for medicines and an amchi's services, in the presence of shifts from barter to cash economies, is also a concern among amchi in Nepal and India. See Besch (2003) and Craig (forthcoming 2004) for more details.

practice remains a key component of their ability to heal and make effective medicines, even if they do not perform healing rituals, as such. As mentioned in Chapter Three, some of these private physicians also purposefully create medicines that conform to their own standards of 'good manufacturing practices': medications are tailor made for individual patients, after careful pulse and urine analysis, and are sometimes even ground on-site or given unground to patients, who take the compounds home and grind the medicine themselves. In addition, such renowned *amchi* are also able to circumvent some of the problems to do with supply of medicinal raw materials and economic survival. Local patients, as well as some patients who travel from great distances to seek out treatment, will come bearing offerings of medicinal ingredients. Sometimes *amchi* will request that people collect specific ingredients for them. In addition, such *amchi* rarely if ever ask for payment for their services. A traditional sense of reciprocity prevails: patients of varying economic means make offerings in cash and kind to such healers, while the poorest patients are not expected to offer any payment. Some of these private practice physicians maintain links to state *sowa rigpa* institutions, while others do not. Many such healers have a constant stream of patients, sometimes even more than the local hospital or clinic. In addition, other kinds of healers – from spirit mediums and oracles to lamas – continue to provide patients with other kinds of treatments, such as protective amulets and a variety of ritual blessings, *chinlab*. As mentioned in Chapter Two, such private and primarily lineage-based *amchi* also continue to teach students on a limited basis.

When asked about the presence of such private practice *amchi* in Tibet's contemporary social context, one well-educated urban Tibetan responded: *Maybe people who still practice only sowa rigpa and who do it in the old ways still exist in some places. There aren't any in my home village, though. Maybe there are still some monks or other learned people who know medicine in this way and who practice in some monasteries or in their homes. But those people are more like healers than doctors, more like lamas than scientists.*

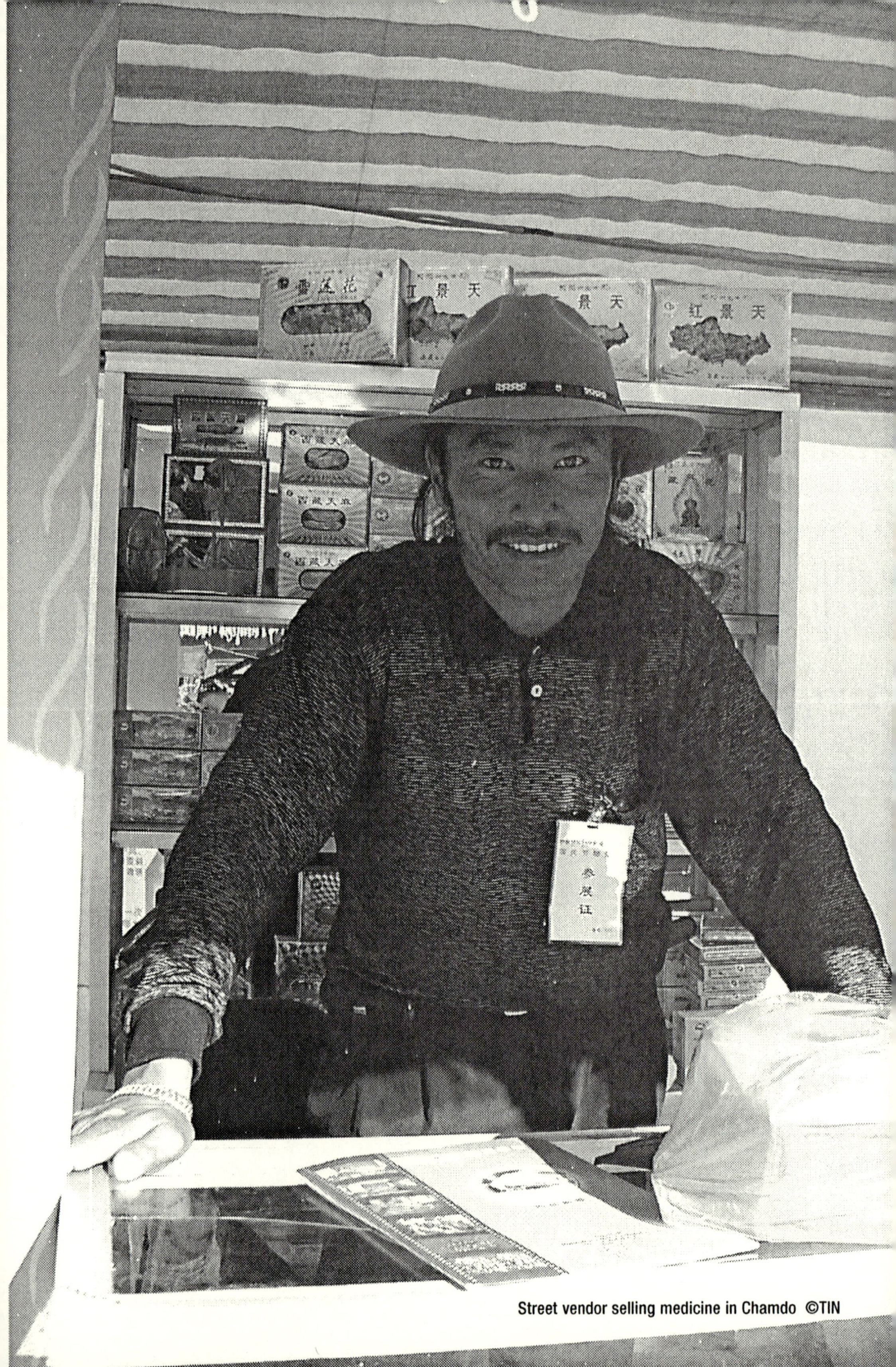

Street vendor selling medicine in Chamdo ©TIN

Conclusion: 'Traditional' Tibetan Medicine and the 'Modern' World

This discussion of the history, present circumstances, and future of Tibetan medicine in contemporary Tibet has raised a range of issues and concerns. We have framed this account of Tibetan medicine today with some historical and religious background. We have examined shifts in how medical and cultural knowledge is being passed from generation to generation, including pressures to standardise this diverse system of oral and literary scholarship and practice. We have addressed the historical and contemporary production of Tibetan medicines themselves, and the growing Tibetan pharmaceutical industry, as well as the effects this industry is having – and threatens to have – on the Tibetan landscape. We have also discussed some of the impacts of government health policies and NGO funding priorities on the health of rural and urban Tibetan communities. Finally, we have explored the relationship between Tibetan medicine and biomedicine in the realm of clinical practice. Now, in conclusion, we turn to some of the larger themes and questions that have surfaced through these chapters.

As a place to begin, consider the following passages, taken from a PRC governmental report on medical service in Tibet:[32]

> *"A total of 32 Tibetan medicine works have been compiled and published; 13 out of 26 scientific research projects won technological progress awards at the regional or ministerial level. Ranmasnagpei, a Traditional Tibetan Medicinal drug, won international awards two times; and another Tibetan medicine named Zotai won the State patent (...) Up till now, the TAR has 14 drugs listed in the State Medical Code; 41 kinds of Tibetan medicinal herbs and 97 Tibetan medicine drugs listed in the standard Tibetan medicine drugs of the Ministry of Public Health; 35 kinds of Tibetan medicine drugs and preparations listed into the standard Tibetan medicine drugs. All these pave way for Tibetan medicine to expand Chinese and foreign market shares...[In] October 1997, the people's government of the TAR held its second congress on Tibetan medicine. The conference made the decision on Strengthening Tibetan Medicine Work, and adopted the Ninth Five-Year Plan on Tibetan Medicine Cause (1996-2000) and the Plan for Further Development in the 2000-2010 Period. The participants agreed that the production of Tibetan medicine should adapt to the market economic structural reform. While maintaining the characteristic of Tibetan medicine, efforts should be made to combine clinical treatment with scientific research, and combine Tibetan medicine with traditional Chinese medicine and Western medicine. Only In this way can Tibetan medicine develop further."*

32 Yun (1999)

This excerpt from a government publication on Tibetan medicine encapsulates many of the forces at work in transforming, supporting, and placing at risk *sowa rigpa* knowledge and practice in Tibetan areas of the PRC and beyond. Namely: the drive to profit from Tibetan medicines as well as to make them available as one choice among many in the national and global health care market; the value placed on standardisation of medicines and medical practices, sometimes at the expense of private practitioners and poor communities; the emphasis on 'integrating' Tibetan medicine with biomedicine (and, in the case of the PRC, Traditional Chinese Medicine as well); and the pressure to keep up the image of Tibetan medicine as 'traditional'.

Many of the challenges to the survival of Tibetan culture within the PRC have everything to do with Tibet's recent history and the impacts of Chinese political, social and economic control, as well as the more general trends shaping the modern Chinese state. After the Cultural Revolution, for instance, persecution of aspects of Tibetan medicine deemed suspect by the government was replaced by a period of secularist reforms that have ultimately had a much more lasting influence on the history and practice of Tibetan medicine. As Vincanne Adams has written, this period has been marked by several trends:

> *The first is the marriage of an existing socialist materialism with an uncritical importation of Western-based scientific technologies believed to guarantee rapid and uniform modernisation. This marriage was carried out as a political mandate within the health system. In contrast, the second trend has entailed efforts to revitalise specific traditional cultural practices, including selected religious practices that were no longer believed to threaten the materialist foundations of the nation. The merging of these two trends in Tibet has led on the one hand to a great nostalgia and reverence for the minority cultures on the part of Han majorities and on the other hand to a fragile sense of security concerning the legitimacy of traditional cultural practices among Tibetans themselves. Increasingly, the minorities are seen as resources for recuperating the lost cultural treasures of the greater Chinese nation, and even Tibet medical practitioners are overtly compelled to join the effort to sustain and revitalise their traditional practices. At the same time, the terms of Tibetan involvement in this project are constantly sources of self-questioning because they are labelled as potential sites of political dissent.*[33]

In other words, the Chinese annexation of Tibet has had many lasting effects on Tibetan medical practice – effects that are felt to this day and that will shape the future of *sowa rigpa* inside the PRC. However, many of the changes facing Tibetan medicine in China are also at work among exile communities in India, Nepal and the West. It might even be concluded that the challenges for Tibetan medicine in general are increased in Tibet itself. As a result, sooner or later the other communities practicing Tibetan medicine will be challenged in the same manner. There is sometimes a tendency to view Tibetan medicine as it is practiced in Tibetan areas of the PRC today as a fundamentally

33 Adams (1999:4-5)

compromised iteration of *sowa rigpa*, given the political circumstances of Tibet and Tibetans within the PRC. As we have explored, at different points in Tibet's recent history, overtly 'religious' or ritualistic aspects of Tibetan medical practice have been distinguished from those practices more easily aligned with 'science'; sometimes these practices have been blatantly persecuted. However, it would be a mistake to conclude that *amchi* who treat both through the dispensation of medicines and through healing rituals or the production of ritual blessing medicines are no longer found in Tibet, that 'pure' or 'traditional' Tibetan medicine, in this sense, only exists within the Tibetan exile community, or that *only* Tibetans medical practitioners within the PRC are facing pressures in the realm of medical education, medicine production, or clinical practice. Indeed, a survey of the landscape on both sides of the Himalayas reveals a number of quite similar social, political and economic forces of change coming to bear on Tibetan medicine, not the least of which is the pharmaceutical industry – an iteration of global market forces that includes the commoditisation of disease and the pharmacologisation of health care.

At a certain level, Tibetan investment (both social and financial) in Tibetan medical research can be understood as a necessary response by *sowa rigpa* practitioners to demands placed on traditional practices in today's world. Research efforts, like battles over Intellectual Property Rights (IPRs), can be justified as a way of safeguarding ethnomedicine and the genius of indigenous knowledge in the contemporary context. Yet the question that remains is how to conceive of modern Tibetan life in a way that neither denigrates Tibetan cultural practices, including Tibetan medicine, as 'backwards' nor confines *sowa rigpa* to the static realm of 'tradition' without the capacity for invention and change.

When we begin to examine this transformation of *sowa rigpa* and concomitant challenges to Tibetan worldviews, we are confronted with a number of issues that are *not* unique to Tibetan areas of the PRC. The forces working to transform Tibetan medicine are both internal and external. Some are cynical or derive from a motivation toward profit, greed, social and political control and environmental exploitation. Others are well-intentioned efforts to bridge systems of knowledge, keep this aspect of Tibetan culture alive and seek relief from suffering for human communities. Most fall somewhere in the middle. Again, these stresses are not only a product of China's annexation of Tibet. Often, they have much more to do with the structural elements of hegemonic power (either western or Chinese varieties) and the assumptions about 'science' and 'progress' that have informed our conceptions of humanitarian aid and development, or the use of natural resources within a capitalist economy, than they do the specifics of Tibet's political, social and economic position vis-à-vis China.

Finally, it is important to stress that a more equal balance of power – and a true sense of collaboration – between and across cultures and medical systems is possible. People are actively pursuing such collaborations across the globe: western scientists and biomedical practitioners, *amchi*, Buddhist teachers, development workers, anthropologists, botanists, patients, etc.

The Dalai Lama made the following comments in a recent public message on the occasion of the Second International Congress of Tibetan Medicine, held in Washington DC in November 2003:

> *I have always maintained that Tibetan medicine must be understood on its own terms, as well as in the context of objective scientific investigation…Science is playing an important role in validating and recognising age-old knowledge and practices which were developed by many great sages and wise people of Tibet… I am glad that the meeting will also focus on issues of environmental sustainability of medicinal plants… This is a critical issue which must be addressed by all those interested in using traditional medicine…Today, as we face new and growing difficult times, as well as devastating epidemics and diseases, we must work to find new ways to bring peace and healing to the world. I think some of these 'new' approaches might be found in old, traditional knowledge and wisdom – it is my sincerest hope that Tibetan medicine and Buddhism will make a contribution to the health of all humanity.*

Glossary of Tibetan Terms

Tibetan (Phonetically)	Tibetan	English Translation / Definition
amchi	ཨེམ་ཆི།	Physician, doctor, practitioner of Tibetan medicine
bekhen	བད་ཀན།	'phlegm' humour
Bön	བོན་ཆོས།	Pre-Buddhist religious traditions and practices of Tibet
Bumshi	གསོ་རིག་མདོ་དགུ་འབུམ་བཞི།	Four Medical Tantras according to Bön tradition
chang lug	བྱང་ལུགས།	Northern School of Tibetan medicine (until 17th century)
chagpori	ལྕགས་པོ་རི།	Literally 'Iron Hill'; name of hill in Lhasa for which Tibet's first medical college was named; original school was destroyed in 1959; current school of same name founded in Darjeeling, India, in 1992
chi dar	ཕྱི་དར།	Second dissemination of Buddhism in Tibet (from 10th century)
chi - Nang	ཕྱི་ནང་།	Literally 'inside – outside', a distinction that separates Buddhists from non-Buddhists
chima gyu	ཕྱི་མ་རྒྱུད།	Last Tantra, the fourth volume in the Gyushi
chinlab	བྱིན་རླབས།	Ritual blessing medicine, long life medicine, often given in the form of small rilbu
chipa	བྱིས་པ།	Paediatrics
chu	ཆུ།	Water, river; Tibetan element translated as 'water'
chung wa nga	འབྱུང་བ་ལྔ།	Five elements: earth, air, fire, water, and space/consciousness
do	རྡོ།	General category of stones used in Tibetan medical compounds
dön ne	གདོན་ནད།	Disorders caused by spirits

Tibetan Transliteration	Tibetan	English Translation / Definition
dug	དུག	Toxicology
dug sum	དུག་གསུམ། ༡་འདོད་ཆགས། ༢་ཞེ་སྡང་། ༣་གཏི་མུག	Three poisons (1. attachment, 2. hatred, and 3. desire)
Durapa	བསྲས་ར་བ།	Bachelor's degree in Tibetan medicine
ge	གསོ།	Rejuvenation therapies
gyu	རྒྱུད།	Lineage, tantra, continuum
Gyushi	རྒྱུད་བཞི།	Four Medical Tantras
jigten	འཇིག་རྟེན།	The mundane realm of human rebirth
la dzi	ག་རྩི།	Musk glands used in Tibetan medicine
le	ལས།	The laws of cause and effect; *karma* in Sanskrit
lhapa / lhamo	ལྷ་པ། ལྷ་མོ།	Male/female oracle
lha menpa	ལྷ་སྨན་པ།	Literally 'god physician', title given to physicians of important people, such as His Holiness the Dalai Lama
lu [dp]	ལུས།	The body
lu shung dun	ལུས་ཞུངས་བདུན།	Seven bodily constituents
loong	རླུང་།	'wind' humour; Tibetan element translated as 'air'
mani rilbu	མ་ཎི་རིལ་བུ།	Literally 'prayer pill', these are a type of ritual blessing medicines, often distributed during large public gatherings such as Buddhist teachings
ma rigpa	མ་རིག་པ།	ignorance
me	མེ།	Fire, flame; Tibetan element translated as 'fire'
mendrup	སྨན་སྒྲུབ།	Medical empowerment ritual
menkhang	སྨན་ཁང་།	Literally 'house of medicine', general term for clinic, hospital, or pharmacy, depending on context
menpa	སྨན་པ།	Physician, doctor, practitioner of Tibetan medicine
men ngag	མན་ངག	Oral tantric medicine rituals

Tibetan Transliteration	Tibetan	English Translation / Definition
men ngag gyu		Oral Instruction Tantra, the third volume in the Gyushi
Mentsikhang Men-tsee-khang		'House of Medicine and Astrology'
mi rig		Class, race, or category of humans; 'nationality' in the PRC context; *minzu* in Chinese
mo nay		Gynaecology
nam kha		Space, sky; Tibetan element translated as 'space/consciousness'
nga dar		First dissemination of Buddhism in Tibet (7th – 9th centuries)
ngo		General category of herbs used in Tibetan medical compounds
nyepa sum		Three humours; literally 'three faults/illnesses/imbalances'
rilbu		Tibetan medicine pill
rinchen rilbu		Precious pills
rinpoche		Literally 'precious jewel', honorific title given to Tibetan religious masters; general category of precious and semi-precious stones and gems used in Tibetan medicinal compounds
ro drug		Six tastes
ro tsa		Aphrodisiac therapies
sa		Earth, soil, land; the Tibetan element translated as 'earth'; general category of soils used in Tibetan medical compounds
Sangye Menla		Medicine Buddha; literally 'Master of Remedies'
sem		Literally 'heart-mind'
ser khab		Golden needle acupuncture
Shang Shung		Ancient western Tibetan kingdom
shey gyu		Explanatory Tantra, the second volume in the Gyushi
shib jug		Research
sog chag		General category of animal products used in Tibetan medical compounds

Tibetan Transliteration	Tibetan	English Translation / Definition
sog loong	སྲོག་རླུང་།	Literally 'life force wind humour', when out of balance associated with depression, anxiety, and other mental illness
so rig lab dra chenmo	བོད་སློང་ས་གསོ་རིག་སློབ་གྲྭ་ཆེན་མོ།	Tibetan Medical College
sowa rigpa	གསོ་བ་རིག་པ།	Tibetan medicine; Tibet's 'science of healing'
sugpo	གཟུགས་པོ།	Corporeal body
sur lug	བྱུར་ལུགས།	Southern School of Tibetan medicine (until 17th century)
terma	གཏེར་མ།	Treasures in the form of texts or relics that are hidden by Buddhist masters and revealed at appropriate times.
thang	ཐང་།	General category of shrubs used in Tibetan medical compounds
thangka	ཐང་ག	Tibetan-style scroll painting
tripa	མཁྲིས་པ།	'bile' humour
tsa loong	རྩ་རླུང་།	Literally 'channel wind', relates to circulation and a particular group of meditation instructions
tsenpo	བཙན་པོ།	Title given to lineage of rulers during the Tibetan imperial period (7th – 9th century) originally from the Yarlung Valley region east of Lhasa
tsa gyu	རྩ་རྒྱུད།	Root Tantra, the first volume in the Gyushi
tsön	མཚོན།	Trauma wounds
tsi	རྩི།	General category of mucilaginous substances used in Tibetan medical compounds
wang	དབང་།	Empowerment; power
yartsa gunbu	དབྱར་རྩ་དགུན་འབུ།	Literally 'summer grass winter insect', *cordyceps sinensis*

Bibliography

Adams, V. (1999). Equity of the Ineffable: Cultural and Political Constraints on Ethnomedicine as a Health Problem in Contemporary Tibet. Foundations of Health and Equity, Harvard Centre for Population and Development Studies.

Adams, V. (2000a). Complications in the Study of Efficacy of Tibetan Medicine within the Biomedical Context. International Academic Conference on Tibetan Medicine, Lhasa, TAR, PRC.

Adams, V. (2000b). "Women's Health in Tibetan Medicine and Tibet's 'First' Female Doctor." Women's Buddhism, Buddhism's Women: Tradition, Revision, Renewal. E. B. Findly, ed. Cambridge, MA: Wisdom Publications, 433-450.

Adams, V. (2001a). Particularizing Modernity: Tibetan Medical Theorizing of Women's Health in Lhasa, Tibet. Healing Powers and Modernity: Traditional Medicine, Shamanism, and Science in Asian Societies. L. H. Connor and G. Samuel. Westport, CT and London, Bergin and Garvey.

Adams, V. (2001b). "The Sacred in the Scientific: Ambiguous Practices of Science in Tibetan Medicine." Cultural Anthropology 16(4): 542-575.

Adams, V. (2002a). Establishing Proof: Translating "Science" and the State in Tibetan Medicine. New Horizons in Medical Anthropology: Essays in Honour of Charles Leslie. M. Nichter and. M. Lock, eds. London and New York, Routledge: 200-220.

Adams, V. (2002b). "Randomised Controlled Crime: Postcolonial Sciences in Alternative Medicine Research." Social Studies of Science 32(5-6): 1-32.

Adams, V. (2003). "The Cross-Cultural Challenge in Clinical Trials Research." Paper presented at the Second International Congress on Tibetan Medicine, Washington DC, November 5-8, 2003.

Adams, V. and F. F. Li (forthcoming 2004). "Integration or Erasure: Modernization at the Mentsikhang." Tibetan Medicine in Contemporary Context. L. Pordie, ed London and New Delhi: Routledge

van Alphen, J. and A. Aris, Eds. (1995). Oriental Medicine: An Illustrated Guide to the Asian Arts of Healing. London, Serindia Publications.

Aschoff, J. (1996). Annotated Bibliography of Tibetan Medicine (1789-1995). Ulm/Germany: Fabri Verlag and Dietikon/Switzerland: Garuda Verlag.

Baker, I. (1997). The Tibetan Art of Healing. San Francisco, Chronicle Books.

Beckwith, C. I. (1979). "The Introduction of Greek Medicine into Tibet in the Seventh and Eighth Centuries." Journal of the American Oriental Society 99(2): 297-313.

Besch, F. (2003). "Professionalisation among *amchi* in Spiti: discussing the modernization of Tibetan medicine." Paper presented at the Tibetan Medicine Panel of the 10th Annual International Association of Tibetan Studies Conference, St. Hugh's College, Oxford University, Oxford, England, September 6-12,2003.

Birnbaum, R. (1989). The Healing Buddha. Boston, MA, Shambhala.

Bradley, T. (2000). Principles of Tibetan Medicine. London: Thorson's/HarperCollins Publishers.

Burang, T. (1974). Tibetan Art of Healing. London, Robinson and Watkins Books Ltd.

Chen, C.C. (1989). Medicine in Rural China. Berkeley: University of California Press.

Clark, B. (1995). The Quintessence Tantras of Tibetan Medicine. Ithaca, NY, Snow Lion.

Clifford, T. (1984). Tibetan Buddhist Medicine and Psychiatry. York Beach, ME, Samuel Weiser.

Craig, S. (1998). Portrait of a Himalayan Healer. Explorer's Journal. 1998.

Craig, S. (forthcoming 2004). "Place and Professionalisation: Navigating *amchi* identity in Nepal," in L. Pordie, ed. Tibetan Medicine in Contemporary Context. London and New Delhi: Routledge.

Crow, D. (2000). In Search of the Medicine Buddha: A Himalayan Journey. New York, Tarcher Putnam.

Crozier, R. (1968). Traditional Medicine in Modern China. Cambridge, MA: Harvard University Press.

Dash, V. B. (1976). Tibetan Medicine with Special Reference to Yoga Sataka. Dharamsala, Library of Tibetan Works and Archives.

Dash, V. B. (1994). Pharmacopoeia of Tibetan Medicine. Delhi, Sri Satguru Publications.

Dawa, Dr., (1999). A Clear Mirror of Tibetan Medicinal Plants. Rome: Tibet Domani

Dhonden, Y. D. (1986). Health Through Balance. Ithaca, Snow Lion.

Dhonden, Y. D. (2000). Healing from the Source: The Science and Lore of Tibetan Medicine. Ithaca, NY, Snow Lion Publications.

Dorje, Gawo, et. al, eds. (1995). *'khrungs dpe dri med shel gyi me long* / The Clear Pure Mirror: A Compendium of the Development of Tibetan Materia Medica. Lhasa, Tibet: mi rigs dpe skrun khang / People's Publishing House.

Dummer, T. (1988). Tibetan Medicine and Other Holistic Health-Care Systems. London, Routledge.

Ernst, Waldrud, (2002). 'Plural Medicine, Tradition, and Modernity: Historical and

Contemporary Perspectives: Views from Below and Above.' W. Ernst, ed. Plural Medicine, Tradition, and Modernity, 1800 – 2000. London: Routledge.

Farquhar, Judith, (1994). Knowing Practice: the Clinical Encounter of Chinese Medicine. Boulder, CO, Westview Press, 1994.

Fenton, P. (1999). Tibetan Healing: The Modern Legacy of Medicine Buddha. Wheaton, IL and

Chennai(Madras), India, Quest Books.

Finckh, E. (1988). Studies in Tibetan Medicine. Ithaca, NY, Snow Lion.

Gerke, Barbara, ed. (1997-2002). Ayur Vijnana: A Periodical on Indo-Tibetan and Allied Medical Cultures. Kalimpong, India: International Trust for Tibetan Medicine, volumes 1-8.

Gerke, Barbara and Eric Jacobson, (1996). 'Traditional Asian Medical Cultures Encounter Biomedical Research.' Ayur Vijnana, Kalimpong, India, International Trust for Traditional Medicine, vol. 1.

Gerke, B. (1999). "On the history of the two Tibetan medical schools Janglug and Zurlug". Ayur Vijnana: A Periodical on Indo-Tibetan and Allied Medical Cultures. Kalimpong: International Trust for Traditional Medicine. (6): 17-25.

Gerke, B. (2003). "A Brief History of Tibetan Medicine." Article prepared for the Wellcome Trust, London, UK.

Gyatso, J. (1993). "The Logic of Legitimation in the Tibetan Treasure Tradition," History of Religions. 33(2): 97-134.

Gyatso, J. (2003). "Mapping the body with Buddhism: shifting fortunes of the tantric channel system in Tibetan medical anatomy." Tibetan Medicine Panel of the 10th Annual International Association of Tibetan Studies Conference, St. Hugh's College, Oxford University, Oxford, England, September 6-12,2003.

Institute for High Plateau Plant Research of Chinese Academy of Sciences, eds, (1996). *bod sman gyi rnam bshas* / Introduction to Tibetan Medicine. Xining: Qinghai People's Publishing House.

Jamison, D., J. Evans, T. King, I. Porter, N. Prescott, and A. Proust (1984). China: The health sector. Washington DC: The World Bank.

Janes, C. (1995). "The Transformations of Tibetan Medicine." Medical Anthropology Quarterly 9(1): 6-39.

Janes, C. (1999a). "The health transition and the crisis of traditional medicine: The case of Tibet Social Science and Medicine. 48:1803-1820.

Janes, C. (1999b). "Imagined lives, suffering and the work of culture: The embodied discourses of conflict in modern Tibet. Medical Anthropology Quarterly. 13: 391-412.

Janes, C. (2001). Tibetan Medicine at the Crossroads: Radical Modernity and the Social Organization of Traditional Medicine in the Tibet Autonomous Region, China. Healing Powers and Modernity: Traditional Medicine, Shamanism, and Science in Asian Societies. L. H. Connor and G. Samuel. Westport, CT and London, Bergin and Garvey.

Kapstein, M. (2000). The Tibetan Assimilation of Buddhism: Conversion, Contestation, and Memory. Oxford and New Delhi: Oxford University Press.

Khangkar, D. (1998). Tibetan medicine: The Buddhist Way of Healing. New Delhi, Lustre Press Pvt. Ltc., Roli Books.

Kletter, C. and M. Kriechbaum, Eds. (2001). Tibetan Medicinal Plants. Boca Raton, London, New York, and Washington DC, Medpharm Scientific Publishers.

Lama, Yeshi, et al., (2001). Medicinal Plants of Dolpo: Amchis' Knowledge and\Conservation. Kathmandu, Nepal, World Wildlife Fund Nepal Programme Publication Series, 2001.

Library of Tibetan Works and Archives. (1981-1992). Tibetan Medicine Series 1-11.

McKay, A. (2003). "Himalayan medical encounters: the establishment of Western biomedicine in Tibet." Paper presented at the Tibetan Medicine Panel of the 10th Annual International Association of Tibetan Studies Conference, St. Hugh's College, Oxford University, Oxford, England, September 6-12, 2003.

Men-tsee-khang (2001). Fundamentals of Tibetan Medicine. Dharamsala, Men-tsee-khang (Tibetan Medical and Astrological Institute of HH the Dalai Lama).

Mentsikhang (2002). The Native Land of Traditional Tibetan Medicine (Brochure). Lhasa, TAR, PRC, Mentsikhang (Tibetan Medical Hospital and Factory of the TAR).

Meyer, F. (1983). GSO-BA RIGPA: Le Systéme médical tibetain. Paris, Editions du Centre National de Recherche Scientifique.

Meyer, F. (1981). Gso-ba-rig-pa, Le systeme medical tibétain, Paris: Presses du CNRS.

Meyer, F. (1995). Theory and Practice of Tibetan Medicine. Oriental Medicine: An Illustrated Guide to the Asian Arts of Healing. J. van Alphen and F. Meyer., eds. London, Serendia.

Meyer, F. (1995). Tibetan Medicine Today: A View from Outside Tibet. Oriental Medicine: An Illustrated Guide to the Asian Arts of Healing. J. van Alpen and F. Meyer. London, Serendia.

Meyer, F. (1998). The History and Foundations of Tibetan Medicine. The Buddha's Art of Healing: Tibetan Paintings Rediscovered. John F. Avedon, ed. New York, Rizzoli.

Millard, C. (2002). Learning Processes in a Tibetan Medical School. PhD. Dissertation. University of Edinburgh, Department of Social Anthropology.

Millard, C. (2003). "The adaptation of Tibetan medicine in a Western Cultural Context." Paper presented at the Tibetan Medicine Panel of the 10th Annual International Association of Tibetan Studies Conference, St. Hugh's College, Oxford University, Oxford, England, September 6-12,2003.

Namdrul, T. (2003). "Tibetan medicine in the 21st Century: a clinical trial of Tibetan medicine in the treatment of newly diagnosed non-insulin dependent diabetes mellitus (NIDDM). Paper presented at the Tibetan Medicine Panel of the 10th Annual International Association of Tibetan Studies Conference, St. Hugh's College, Oxford University, Oxford, England, September 6-12,2003.

Parfionovitch, Y., and G. Dorje, et al., Eds. (1992). Tibetan Medical Paintings: Illustrations to the Blue Beryl Treatise of Sangye Gyamtso (1653-1705). London, Serindia Publications.

Pordie, L. (2002). "Pharmacopoeia as an Expression of Society: A Himalayan Study." From the Roots of Knowledge to Future Medicines. Fleurentin *et al*. eds. Paris: Publ. French Society for Ethnopharmacology – Research Institute for Development.

Rapgay, L. (1984). Tibetan Medicine: A holistic approach to better health. Dharamsala, India, Tibet Medical and Astrological Institute.

Rapgay, L. (2000). The Tibetan Book of Healing. Northampton, MA: Lotus Publishers.

Rechung, R. (1973). Tibetan Medicine. London, Wellcome Institute of the History of Medicine.

Schwabl, H. (2003). "Issues of Quality Control for Tibetan Medicinal Products." Paper presented at the Second International Congress on Tibetan Medicine, Washington DC, November 5-8, 2003.

Sachs, R., Gyaltsen, D. and L. Rapgay. (2001). Tibetan Ayurveda: Health Secrets from the Roof of the World. Inner Traditions International, Ltd.

Sarah Sallon, et al, 2003. *Mercury in Traditional Tibetan Medicine: Problem or Panacea?* Paper given at the Second International Congress on Tibetan Medicine, Washington DC, November 5 - 8, 2003.

Samel, G. (2001). Tibetan Medicine. London: Little Brown UK.

Samuel, G. (1993). Civilized Shamans: Buddhism in Tibetan Societies. Kathmandu: Mandala Book Point.

Samuel, G. (1999). "Religion, Health, and Suffering among Contemporary Tibetans." Religion, Health, and Suffering. J. Hinnell and R. Porter, eds. London and New York: Kegan Paul International.

Samuel, G. (2001). Tibetan Medicine in Contemporary India: Theory and Practice. Healing Powers and Modernity: Traditional Medicine, Shamanism, and Science in Asian Societies. L. H. Connor and G. Samuel. Westport, CT and London, Bergin and Garvey.

Snellgrove, D. and H. Richardson (1995). A Cultural History of Tibet. Boston: Shambhala Publications.

Tsarong, T. J. (1986). Handbook of Traditional Tibetan Drugs. Kalimpong, India, Tibetan Medical Publications.

Tsarong, T. J. (1994). Tibetan Medical Plants. Kalimpong, India, Tibetan Medical Publications.

Unkrig, W.A. (1953), "An Introduction" Die Tibetische Medizinphilosophie (Philosophy of Tibetan Medicine). P. Cyrill von Korvin-Krasinski, ed. Zürich. Translated from the German by B. Gerke and reprinted in *Ayur Vijnana* (8)2002: 9-27.

Xu, X. (1997). "National Essence" vs. "Science": Chinese Native Physicians' Fight for Legitimacy, 1913 – 1937. Modern Asian Studies. (31): 4: 847-877.

Young, M. E. (1989). "Impact of the rural reform on financing rural health services in China." Health Policy. 11(1989): 27-42.

Yun, Z. (1999). Medicare Service in Tibet. Tibet Series. Lhasa, TAR, PRC, China Intercontinental Press: 19-24.

Suggestions for Readers with a General Interest in Tibetan Medicine

Adams, V. (2002). "Randomised Controlled Crime: Postcolonial Sciences in Alternative Medicine Research." Social Studies of Science 32(5-6): 1-32.

van Alphen, J. and A. Aris, eds. (1995). Oriental Medicine: An Illustrated Guide to the Asian Arts of Healing. London, Serindia Publications.

Baker, I. (1997). The Tibetan Art of Healing. San Francisco, Chronicle Books.

Birnbaum, R. (1989). The Healing Buddha. Boston, MA, Shambhala.

Clark, B. (1995). The Quintessence Tantras of Tibetan Medicine. Ithaca, NY, Snow Lion.

Clifford, T. (1984). Tibetan Buddhist Medicine and Psychiatry. York Beach, ME, Samuel Weiser.

Crow, D. (2000). In Search of the Medicine Buddha: A Himalayan Journey. New York, Tarcher Putnam.

Dawa, Dr. (1999). A Clear Mirror of Tibetan Medicinal Plants. Rome: Tibet Domani.

Dhonden, Y. D. (1986). Health Through Balance. Ithaca, Snow Lion.

Dhonden, Y. D. (2000). Healing from the Source: The Science and Lore of Tibetan Medicine. Ithaca, NY, Snow Lion Publications.

Dummer, T. (1988). Tibetan Medicine and Other Holistic Health-Care Systems. London, Routledge.

Fenton, P. (1999). Tibetan Healing: The Modern Legacy of Medicine Buddha. Wheaton, IL and Chennai(Madras), India, Quest Books.

Janes, C. R. (1995). "The Transformations of Tibetan Medicine." Medical Anthropology Quarterly 9(1): 6-39.

Men-tsee-khang (2001). Fundamentals of Tibetan Medicine. Dharamsala, Men-tsee-khang (Tibetan Medical and Astrological Institute of HH the Dalai Lama).

Meyer, F. (1998). The History and Foundations of Tibetan Medicine. The Buddha's Art of Healing: Tibetan Paintings Rediscovered. John F. Avedon, ed. New York, Rizzoli.

Parfionovitch, Y., and G. Dorje, et al., Eds. (1992). Tibetan Medical Paintings: Illustrations to the Blue Beryl Treatise of Sangye Gyamtso (1653-1705). London, Serindia Publications.

Rapgay, L. (2000). The Tibetan Book of Healing. Northampton, MA: Lotus Publishers.

Rechung, R. (1973). Tibetan Medicine. London, Wellcome Institute of the History of Medicine.

Sachs, R., Gyaltsen, D., and L. Rapgay. (2001). Tibetan Ayurveda: Health Secrets from the Roof of the World. Inner Traditions International, Ltd.

9 780954 196172